Typhoid and the Politics of Public Health in Nineteenth-Century Philadelphia

.

Typhoid and the Politics of Public Health in Nineteenth-Century Philadelphia

Michael P. McCarthy

American Philosophical Society
Independence Square   Philadelphia
1987

Memoirs
of the
American Philosophical Society
Held at Philadelphia
For Promoting Useful Knowledge
Volume 179

Library of Congress Catalog Card No. 86-72881
International Standard Book No.: 0-87169-179-5
US ISSN: 0065-9738

Contents

List of Plates   vii
Preface   ix
Introduction   1
I. A Question of Options   5
II. Reformers in Charge   18
III. The Road toward Consensus   41
IV. A Victory for the Machine   62
V. Construction and More Controversy   84
Index   100

List of Plates

Plate   1. Map of pumping stations.

Plate   2. Fairmount water works in 1876.

Plate   3. Forebay of Fairmount water works around 1870.

Plate   4. Fairmount water works in the 1890s.

Plate   5. Engine House at Fairmount in the 1890s.

Plate   6. Spring Garden water works in the 1890s.

Plate   7. Spring Garden reservoir at 26th and Master streets
          in the 1890s.

Plate   8. Second section of the East Park reservoir.

Plate   9. Pond and old water works at Germantown
          in the 1890s.

Plate 10. Reservoir at Chestnut Hill in 1890s.

Plate 11. Pumping station at Roxborough in 1890s.

Plate 12. Filter beds under construction at Lower
          Roxborough in 1901.

Plate 13. Interior of filter beds under construction at Lower
          Roxborough filters.

Plate 14. The tunnel of Torresdale conduit during
          construction in 1904.

Plate 15. Filter beds under construction at Torresdale.

Plate 16. Laying pipe at Torresdale around 1904.

Preface

This is the story of how Philadelphia got safe drinking water—or safe so far as the medical standards of the time were concerned, the major culprit in the nineteenth century being typhoid. Today we are no longer quite so confident about our water, knowing that chemical waste from industrial plants poses a new threat—an irony since the chemical chlorine helped greatly to eliminate the danger of typhoid contamination. We know also now that even brand-new plumbing fixtures can poison our water if lead solder is used in violation of building codes, as apparently it was in many homes in the Philadelphia area according to a recent investigation. In short, safe is relative, and in the years examined here, it meant free from bacteriological infection.

The research for this study relied heavily on the special resources of several area libraries, and I would like to thank the Philadelphia City Archives, the Germantown Historical Society, Bryn Mawr College, Haverford College, the University of Pennsylvania, Temple University, the College of Physicians, the Library Company of Philadelphia, the American Philosophical Society, the Historical Society of Pennsylvania—and in particular the staffs in the government publications room and newspaper room of the Free Library of Philadelphia at Logan Square where I spent many hours. I would also like to thank Roger Lane of Haverford College and my editor at the American Philosophical Society, Carole N. Le Faivre, for their advice and encouragement.

Introduction

On the tenth of February in 1899 bitter cold air swept into Philadelphia and set a new low for the day when the mercury dropped to 6.2 degrees below zero at 7:35 a.m. In the afternoon it began to snow and blow, with winds between thirty-six and forty miles per hour. By the time the storm finally stopped three days later, eighteen inches had fallen, more than in the great blizzard of 1888, an unkind blow from fate considering that the city was already reeling from another typhoid epidemic.

Typhoid. The disease means little to us today since it is no longer a threat to modern cities, but it frightened the urbanizing world of the late nineteenth century.[1] Typhoid is a virulent micro-organism that attacks the intestinal tract. It can be contracted by hand to hand contact or contaminated food, but in most cases the disease spreads when the excreta of an ill person get into the water supply.

The disease is hard-hitting: patients usually experience vomiting and diarrhea that can cause serious dehydration, which in turn can lead to seizures and comas. Fevers as high as 106 degrees also contribute to the complications that in severe cases are fatal. Children were considered more susceptible, but it was by no means only a childhood disease—Wilbur Wright, the aviation pioneer, died in 1912 at forty-five after contracting typhoid from infected shellfish. (His brother Orville survived a bout with typhoid when he was twenty-five and lived until 1948.)

---

[1]Typhoid is still a threat if basic principles of sanitation are not observed. Vaccines developed in the early 1900s help reduce the chance of infection if an outbreak occurs.

Typhoid usually struck hardest in cities that used water from nearby rivers or lakes; the safer ones were those with aqueducts that tapped upcountry sources. In 1899 statistics for eighteen large cities in the United States showed an average death rate per 100,000 of 34, with the highest that year in Pittsburgh (111) which drank river water; the lowest was Detroit (13) which also drank river water, but its figure jumped to 27 the following year. The lowest death rate in major cities around the turn of the century was in Manhattan and the Bronx (15 in 1899) which were served by an aqueduct system.[2]

In Philadelphia the death rate in 1899 was 75, and 948 persons died that year. Typhoid struck every ward in the city—wealthy and poor alike suffered since infected river water made its way through the entire system. In rank order of fatal diseases, tuberculosis and pneumonia claimed more lives (2,818 and 2,424 respectively in 1899), but typhoid killed more Philadelphians under the age of sixteen than childhood threats of the time like diphtheria and croup (94) or scarlet fever (132).[3]

In the epidemic of 1899, Philadelphia public health officials suspected that infected raw sewerage had somehow entered the Schuylkill River above the Queen Lane pumping station in East Falls, because of the large number of typhoid cases in that district. But typhoid increased nearly everywhere, suggesting that the other pumping stations also were getting infected water. New filtration systems had proven their effectiveness against typhoid in other cities by the late 1890s, and in February the common council approved a bill to begin filtration. In March the bill came up for a vote in the select council. (Philadelphia had a bi-cameral legislature until 1919.)

The mayor and the head of the water bureau blessed the bill. The press was also solidly behind it, and so were a host of influential civic and business associations, who even

---

[2]In 1899 well water was used in parts of Brooklyn, Queens, and Staten Island, which had joined New York in 1898. By the early 1900s the entire city received aqueduct water from upstate.
[3]Board of Health, *Annual Report* (1915). Technically by then the board was called a "bureau," but for most of the years under study here, it was a "board" and references will be cited that way for consistency.

formed a City Emergency Water Committee to coordinate their lobbying efforts. Unfortunately the select council killed the bill, the vote of 24-13 being short of the two-thirds majority required for appropriations. The "typhoid thirteen," as the *Public Ledger* called the dissenting councilmen, thus ended any chances for action in that session of the municipal legislature, which was over shortly thereafter.

Thanks to episodes like this in other civic affairs, Philadelphia suffered from a poor reputation around the turn of the century, and in many respects Lincoln Steffens was only reinforcing an existing stereotype when he called the city "corrupt and contented" in his famous article in *McClure's* in 1903 that was reprinted the following year in his best seller *The Shame of the Cities.* Philadelphia was "a disgrace," he said, not only to itself and Pennsylvania "but to the United States and American character."[4] Over the years the "corrupt and contented" image has persisted and taken on a life of its own—something Philadelphia almost feels it must live up to.

This negative view of the city's performance around the turn of the century is still prevalent. In discussing the water works, for example, Sam B. Warner Jr. calls them "inglorious" because they were unable to keep up with demand, and more importantly because the city allowed "private pollution of the rivers to continue unabated," with high typhoid rates as a result.

According to Warner, the water works reflected the "decline in the effectiveness of [Philadelphia's] municipal government" that took place after 1850. Also, he says, it "shows how the city's general culture of privatism stopped a universal public health program short of full realization. Fear of epidemics had created the water system, but once this fear had abated, little or no public support remained to bring the benefits of the new technology to those who could not afford them."[5]

This stiff criticism is not altogether fair because Philadelphia was trying to find ways to provide safe drinking

---

[4]Steffens, *The Shame of the Cities* (New York, 1957; orig. pub., 1904), 134-136.
[5]Warner, *The Private City: Philadelphia in Three Periods of Its Growth* (Philadelphia, 1968), 108-109. The University of Pennsylvania Press published a second edition in 1987. This edition has a new introductory essay by Warner and an updated bibliography of recent books on Philadelphia.

water for all its residents in the second half of the nineteenth century. Improvements were made in sewer systems and water storage in the 1880s and 1890s, for example, and the city explored the possibilities of new water sources before it decided on filtering its existing supply. Filtration was especially controversial, and the bill debated early in 1899 was not the first to be rejected by the councils. Even so, consensus was reached—in fact, it happened that same year when the councils approved funding for filters in September and voters endorsed the decision at a referendum in November.

This study takes another look at the typhoid story—at the people who were trying to solve the public health crisis: the mayor and councilmen, the heads of the water and health departments, the leaders of civic groups, and outside consultants. It also explores the problem of typhoid from the viewpoint of professionals in the emerging field of public health. Typhoid was a difficult disease to detect and control, and not surprisingly medical experts disagreed about the best way to prevent it. In short, this is a complex story that is best begun at the beginning, which means going back to the early years of the Philadelphia water works.[6]

---

[6]The medical side of the story involves physicians more than hospitals. In the dawn of the age of bacteriology, hospitals were often unable to cope with infectious diseases, and they worried about the risks to other patients. As a result nearly all typhoid victims, of all classes, were treated at home.

I. A Question of Options

In the late eighteenth century, well water in Philadelphia was no longer as "sweet-tasting" as it once had been—a condition that was not surprising considering that Philadelphians had been gradually polluting their groundwater for over a century, from the day the first privy was dug in William Penn's "Faire Country Towne" in the year of its founding in 1682. In the 1790s worries about water came to a head when the city was struck by a wave of yellow fever epidemics. The city fathers blamed their wells and decided to seek a new water supply from the nearby Schuylkill River.

Water pollution was not really the culprit because we know now that a small tropical mosquito, the silvery *Stegomyia fasciata*, is the carrier of yellow fever. Apparently those mosquitoes came to Philadelphia on board ships carrying French refugees from revolution-torn Haiti in the early 1890s.[1] In any case, the decision to seek a new water supply was a good one because polluted water was in fact the cause of many illnesses, and the Schuylkill was a splendid new source, a lovely stream that meandered through virgin woodlands before reaching the city, its water pristine, good-tasting and plentiful in supply.

In 1801 the city began to pump water from an intake basin on the river at the foot of Chestnut Street to holding tanks housed in a lovely Roman-looking domed building at Centre Square where City Hall stands today. Attractive as the pump

---

[1]The first outbreak is discussed fully in J.H. Powell, *Bring Out Your Dead; The Great Plague of Yellow Fever in Philadelphia in 1793* (Philadelphia, 1949). Yellow fever epidemics struck other cities in the 1790s, but Philadelphia was the worst hit. For more on the *Stegomyia fasciata*, see David McCullough, *The Path Between the Seas: The Creation of the Panama Canal, 1870-1914* (New York, 1977), 409ff.

house may have been, its holding tanks were too small to meet demand, and the city decided to shift its pumping operation to a new station at Fairmount where a reservoir of much greater capacity was built atop the hill there. This system was in service by the early 1820s. Although only a small fraction of the city homeowners actually had piped water in those days, free water was available at public pumps around the city, and Philadelphia deservedly enjoyed a reputation as one of the healthiest cities in the world.[2] As the city grew, more pumping stations went up along the Schuylkill—at Spring Garden (1844), Roxborough (1866), Belmont in west Fairmount Park (1870), and at Queen Lane south of Wissahickon Creek (1895). Pumping stations were also added on the Delaware, at Kensington (1851) and at Lardner's Point in Frankfort (1877).[3]

Unfortunately, as the city—and region—grew, water quality plummeted. By the 1880s some 350,000 persons lived along the banks of the Schuylkill from Philadelphia to the booming industrial towns nearby, such as Conshohocken and Norristown. The river had become a "natural sewer," William Ludlow, the chief of the Water Bureau, said in his annual report for 1883, "the character of the pollution" being "as diversified as the occupation of the people: sewerage, chemical, wool-washing, dye stuff, butcher and brewery refuse—there is almost nothing lacking."[4]

The worst problem was within the city limits along the industrial corridor in Manayunk. A water bureau investigation in the early 1880s found that over half of the thirty or so mills and factories along the Schuylkill, which at full capacity hired over 2,300 workers, discharged their toilet wastes directly into the river. The city court and board of health stopped the biggest offenders, but a follow-up check found that many of the others, hiring a total of some 800 workers,

---

[2]Nelson M. Blake, *Water for the Cities* (Syracuse, 1956), 18-43, 78-93.
[3]Until 1854 the city of Philadelphia was only two square miles in area and bounded by Vine and South Streets. The water works at Spring Garden and Kensington were built by suburban governments that were abolished when the city and county consolidated in 1854. The new Philadelphia was 130 square miles and has remained the same size since. See my article, "The Philadelphia Consolidation of 1854: A Reappraisal," *Pennsylvania Magazine of History and Biography* 110 (October, 1986), 531-548.
[4]Bureau of Water, *Annual Report* (1883), 46.

were still polluting the river. In addition investigators found that around sixty-five homes and other buildings in Manayunk, including the police station and several saloons, were using flush toilets hooked up to sewers that drained into the river.[5]

The situation was no better on the Delaware River, which was supplying the city with approximately 20 percent of its water. The Kensington works were becoming notorious for the poor quality of water pumped, since the pumping station was more or less surrounded by industry, which insured "its getting the full benefit of all the city sewerage," Ludlow said sarcastically in his 1883 annual report.

He noted that conditions were "much less objectionable" at another pumping station farther up the Delaware at Lardner's Point, but that water, too, was constantly threatened by the city sewerage the tides frequently carried there. The declining water quality worried Philadelphians because typhoid was a growing problem. Since the city began keeping records on the disease in 1861, the official death toll had risen each decade, from 4,357 deaths in 1861-1869, to 4,416 in the 1870s and up to 6,394 in the 1880s.[6]

What could the city do? One possible solution was to use an aqueduct to bring pure water to the city from new sources. At the time aqueducts were enjoying a modest revival in popularity. They certainly were nothing new, the Romans having had some impressive ones in their day, but virtually none had been built since ancient times until the nineteenth century when cities rediscovered their virtues for improving public health.

Aqueduct systems were not undertaken lightly, given the problems in finding an adequate new water supply, the great construction costs, and the headaches involved in gaining approval from all the local governments and property owners at the dam sites and along the right of way of the aqueduct. In fact most cities that adopted them had no other viable options.

The first major city to build an aqueduct in the United

---

[5]Bureau of Water, *Documents related to the pollution of the Schuylkill River* (1893), 36-40. This is a useful collection of reports that cover several decades.
[6]Figures from table in Board of Health, *Annual Report* (1899), 165.

States, for example, was New York, which was surrounded by water it could not drink, located as it was on Manhattan Island in New York harbor, the tidal flow of the Atlantic Ocean salting the Hudson River and Harlem and East Rivers. (The latter were not really rivers at all, but channels that linked Long Island Sound with the Hudson and the ocean.) By the 1820s New York realized that it could no longer rely on the well water on Manhattan Island, and it began to look afar for an adequate new supply.[7]

New York finally chose the Croton River, which was some thirty miles north of the city. Though relatively distant, the river was well above sea level so that the water could reach New York by gravity flow without the need for pumps. A dam was built across the Croton River to create a reservoir, and the engineers kept the aqueduct at uniform grade by spanning valleys with bridges and tunneling through the countryside in some districts. A great stone bridge carried the aqueduct across the Harlem River to Manhattan where a receiving reservoir was built in what is now Central Park.

A distributing reservoir was located farther south on 42nd Street and Fifth Avenue, at the present site of the main branch of the New York Public Library. In those days most New Yorkers lived in lower Manhattan, which was also lower in elevation than 42nd Street, so water from the tall distributing reservoir could be piped to the upper floors of two and three-story buildings without the need for pumps, making the system very efficient indeed. The system officially went into operation on 4 July 1842, the event being marked by ceremonies and speeches.[8]

Boston, more or less in the middle of salt water, adopted the aqueduct system surrounded as it was on three sides by Boston harbor and the brackish Charles River. In the 1840s following New York's example, Boston built its Cochituate aqueduct that took water from Long Pond, some fourteen miles west. As the virtues of upcountry water became clear in improved health statistics, even cities with available river supplies at their doorstep began to adopt the aqueduct idea,

[7]Blake, *Water*, 100ff.
[8]Ibid., 121-171; Charles Lockwood, *Manhattan Moves Uptown* (Boston, 1976), 184-191.

Washington, D.C. and Paris in the 1850s being two notable examples.[9]

An aqueduct was a practical possibility for Philadelphia too, given the large number of good rivers that could reach the city by gravity flow. In fact surveys had been done as early as the 1860s, and in the spring of 1883, with the typhoid situation getting no better, the city councils decided to take another look at possible future supplies. Work began that summer on what turned out to be a four-year project under Rudolph Hering, a highly respected New York civil engineer who had undertaken similar surveys for other cities. His charge was to survey the waters of all rivers and streams in the region that might produce a supply that was pure but also plentiful enough to meet Philadelphia's needs.

Hering's report, like earlier ones, recommended tapping the upper Delaware River at Point Pleasant in rural Bucks County some 30 miles northeast of Philadelphia and building an aqueduct from there to the city. Another possibility was the Perkiomen River northwest of the city, but that river would have to be linked by canal or a supplementary aqueduct with the Lehigh River farther north in order to assure sufficient flow. Hering used a 1875 engineering report as a basis for his cost estimate of $30 million.[10]

Despite its promise, Philadelphians wanted some answers before they acted on the aqueduct option. High costs were only part of the problem—in many respects the major issue was water quality. Would the aqueduct water be guaranteed safe? And exactly what was safe water? Questions like these were raised, so we need to look here more closely at the medical side of the story.

***

As noted earlier, everyone had long suspected a correla-

---

[9]Blake, *Water*, 119-218, 266; David H. Pinkney, *Napoleon III and the Rebuilding of Paris* (Princeton, 1958), ch. v.
[10]Philadelphia City Councils, *Report of the Water Committee on Water Supply* (1892), 36-40. This is a collection of reports which are summarized and quoted in part.

tion between disease and drinking water, but the medical profession was also a long time in proving it. Scientists in the early nineteenth century thought that mineral content was related to water quality, and the standard tests were for the "hardness" and "softness" of the water.[11] By mid-century, a test for organic solids had become the new standard for measuring water quality. This test was more accurate since the cause of typhoid—human waste—was organic.

Unfortunately algae and other harmless vegetable matter like rotting leaves and grass were also organic, which meant that the tests could give very misleading results. In 1859, for example, the chemist for the board of health in Philadelphia bragged about the "remarkable purity" of the Schuylkill in his annual report, the Schuylkill having an average of only 5.34 grains per gallon of organic solids compared to 10.93 grains found in the Croton water supplied to New York City.[12] These figures seemed to say that the Schuylkill water was twice as pure as the Croton, which made no sense since New York in those years had a much lower rate of water-related diseases than Philadelphia.

The problem, of course, was that leaves fall into reservoirs that are deep in the wooded countryside where New York's reservoirs were located, and algae also thrived in the country reservoirs. As a result, New York's water occasionally looked and even tasted unpleasant, but the vegetable matter was harmless. In short, New York's water was a good deal safer than Philadelphia's, statistical inferences notwithstanding.

In the 1860s scientists developed more sophisticated tests that measured pollution based on the amount of nitrogen and albuminoid ammonia, two chemicals found in human waste. To be sure, those chemicals could be found in some harmless matter too, but health departments everywhere began to use the tests to monitor their own water supplies because they were reliable enough and were the best measure available at the time.

In 1880 a major breakthrough in typhoid control took place. Using increasingly powerful microscopes, along with new stains and gelatins, two German scientists working inde-

[11]Blake, *Water*, 248-250.
[12]Board of Health, *Annual Report* (1859), 46.

pendently at long last identified the typhoid bacilli.[13] Unfortunately, the discovery did not have the immediate impact it deserved. The germ theory of disease was not completely accepted despite all the discoveries in bacteriology in the 1870s and 1880s. Many traditionalists were still staunch supporters of the "miasma" school which believed that disease was caused by atmospheric conditions or vapors that rose from filth.

Miasmists were particularly skeptical of the germ theory of typhoid because, while it was now easy enough to identify the bacilli in blood samples of a victim once a physician knew what to look for, it was quite another thing to find typhoid bacilli in any given sample of drinking water. Minute amounts of typhoid microbes could trigger an epidemic, and you would have to be extraordinarily lucky to find typhoid bacilli in a routine test of the water supply. No one had done it, so miasmists could say that the germ theory was unproven despite all the evidence pointing that way. Like the American Tobacco Institute experts who deny the relationship between smoking and lung cancer, the miasmists remained unconvinced. Our rivers might be a little dirty, they said, but not filled with dangerous microbes.[14]

In spring of 1885 the city councils decided to fund a supplementary study which would be conducted by researchers under their direction rather than the water bureau. They did this in part to mollify the vocal physicians of the miasmist school. Many of the councilmen themselves, however, did not believe the germ theory either, and they were also miffed at the chief of the Water Bureau, Ludlow, because they felt he was hurting Philadelphia's image by his critical remarks about the city's water.

Whatever their motives, the councils seem to have made a fair choice in their appointments, naming a team of three highly regarded chemistry professors headed by Professor J.W. Mallet of the University of Virginia. The team took

---

[13]Mazyck P. Ravene, ed., *A Half Century of Public Health* (New York, 1921; Arno reprint edition, 1970), 70-72.
[14]The earliest work on the germ theory of typhoid and its transmission by water was by the English physician William Budd, who wrote in 1839. It was not until the 1850s, with the work of John Snow on cholera, that the contagionist idea gained respectability if not full support.

samples from the city pumping stations and compared them
with samples Mallet had taken in five cities in 1881 as part of
a survey he conducted for the United States Board of
Health. The team judged Philadelphia's water to be somewhere in the middle in the terms of quality compared to
other cities: not as good as Chicago's or New York's but better than that in Baltimore, Boston, and New Orleans. Given
this finding, it was not surprising that the council water committee thought the worries about the city's water were "exaggerated."[15]

But was the city's water satisfactory? A great number of
variables affected quality, and water that might be quite acceptable at one time could be quite polluted at a different
time. As it happened when Mallet and his team took their
samples, the overall quality in both the Schuylkill and Delaware was quite high, so the results while reassuring were not
necessarily reliable.

One critic was Professor Albert R. Leeds of the Stevens
Institute in New Jersey. Leeds had done a chemical analysis
of the rivers for Hering's report, and he questioned the research design used by Mallett. Leeds said, "No plan can be
adopted, more liable to erroneous results, than that of bas-
ing conclusions as to the character of water in flowing
streams upon the testimony of a few isolated analyses."[16]
Leeds pointed to the great variations he found in the fifty-
nine samples he took from the Spring Garden works. One of
the tests he ran was for albuminoid ammonia in which by the
standards of the time a "good" water had zero to .015 parts
per million; "doubtful" from .015 to .020; "bad" from .020
to .030, and "unfit for use" was over .030 parts per million.

After averaging all fifty-nine tests, Leeds said Spring
Garden water got a rating of .015 or a "doubtful," but his
samples on any given day ran from .008 or "good" to .031 or
"unfit for use."[17] To make matters more confusing, twenty-
three of his water samples were below the .015 average and
thirty-one above it, which is to say that in the fifty-nine tests,

[15]The report is reprinted in Board of Health, *Annual Report* (1885); water committee
quote from *Journal of the Select Council* (6 April 1885-25 September 1885), Appendix
No. 88, 134.
[16]Leeds, *Final Report. . .* in Bureau of Water, *Annual Report* (1886), 382.
[17]Ibid., 389.

the average sample of .015 was actually measured only five times. To be sure, his tests showed that the water at Spring Garden was good some of the time, but it was the other times that worried Leeds.

The variations also worried Dr. Charles Cresson, a Philadelphia physician who served as chemist for the board of health. Cresson had introduced the nitrogen and albuminoid ammonia tests in Philadelphia in the 1870s, and he had done a study of water quality on the Schuylkill from 1884 to 1886 to assist Hering and Leeds in their work. At one time or another, water from all three of the pumping stations Cresson sampled had levels of albuminoid ammonia above .030 or "unfit" level. Far from being "continuously wholesome," as some of its defenders claimed, Cresson felt the Schuylkill was more or less a continuous threat.[18]

Given all the evidence against the Schuylkill, the aqueduct idea should have appealed to those who were not happy with the existing water supply. The implications of the recent breakthroughs in bacteriology, however, made Ludlow and others hesitant about endorsing untested waters, however pure they seemed. As Ludlow pointed out, "It has been proved beyond the shadow of a doubt that water which to every sense is pure may be charged with the most active and deadly potency."[19] Leeds was also worried, and he recommended that the upper Delaware be used only if the water quality remained high at the proposed Point Pleasant pumping station. This prospect did not look promising if a letter that appeared in the Philadelphia *Press* in December of 1886 was at all accurate. In any event, it was reprinted in the council records among other testimony when the water committee held a hearing that month on the new water proposals. Signed by a "J.A.F.," the letter said,[20]

It is generally supposed that the water of the upper Delaware is pure and free of adulteration of other streams of less magnitude,

---

[18]Cresson's remarks from correspondence with Leeds and reprinted in pamphlet, *Water Supply of Philadelphia* (1887), 5.
[19]Bureau of Water, *Annual Report* (1884), 65.
[20]*Report of the Water Committee on Water Supply* (1892), 32. Letter cited by Dr. Charles Dulles in an address to the water committee on 9 December 1886 and reprinted along with excerpts of his remarks.

from which it is proposed to draw the future supply for the City. From personal observation, made between Stroudsburg and Port Jervis at intervals during the past fifteen years, I find that there is a noticeable change in the condition of the water, it being less pure than formerly. There are fifteen towns and villages along the Delaware, above the Water Gap, the most populous being the city of Port Jervis, where the drainage from not less than two thousand dwelling and industrial establishments passes into the river. The water is unpalatable, and is not used by those having access to it. The route of a railroad along the river between Port Jervis and Stroudsburg has been surveyed, and in all probability will be built in the near future. With it would come an increase in the number of industrial establishments and other sources of pollution to the river, which the City of Philadelphia could not prevent. During the months of July and August, thousands of female shad, which expire after spawning, float down the river; and during the past summer I saw the shores lined with their bodies in various stages of decomposition. Although to the eye the water of the upper Delaware is usually quite clear and transparent, it is perhaps not much purer than other proposed sources nearer home.

In light of all the uncertainties and disagreements, it is not surprising that the councils did not take any action on the Hering report. But they did take action on trying to clean the Schuylkill with a major sewer project on the east bank of the river from Manayunk to a discharge point below the Fairmount Dam. Into this "interceptor" sewer were to flow factory and house drains, and street sewer lines of Manayunk, lower Roxborough, and East Falls, communities that were considered to be the worst source of pollution to the Schuylkill water. Work began in the late 1880s and continued into the 1890s with an additional interceptor sewer along the Wissahickon creek. The new sewers probably helped most the Queen Lane pumping station that was just below the outfall of the Wissahickon, but they also helped to cut the pollution at Belmont, Spring Garden, and Fairmount.

The city fathers also agreed on building bigger reservoirs as a way of fighting the pollution problem. Bigger reservoirs meant that water could settle longer before it went to the home faucet. The longer the wait, the clearer the water as dirt particles sank to the bottom, in what was known as the sedimentation process. Experiments also showed that there was an approximate fall-off of 15 percent in the bacteria count of water that "rested" in reservoirs for a forty-eight hour period. This was not a particularly impressive figure even in those days, but it was an improvement nonetheless.

As part of this program, two more reservoirs were added at Roxborough that dramatically increased capacity there— from 12.8 million to 147 million gallons. Another was the East Park reservoir in Fairmount Park north of Girard Avenue and west of 33rd Street, completed in 1892. It was the biggest of the new reservoirs and held around 300 million gallons. East Park and the others gave the city a total storage capacity of 869 million gallons at a time when the city was consuming around 140 million a day. In theory at least this meant that Philadelphia water should have rested in a reservoir for at least forty-eight hours. Unfortunately it did not work that way because some of the reservoirs were not connected, and some of the older reservoirs were quite small in capacity compared to demand.

In 1889, for example, the reservoir in Mount Airy had a capacity of approximately 4.5 million gallons and pumped 2.5 million gallons daily to 35,000 residents in parts of Germantown, Chestnut Hill, Tioga, and a few other nearby neighborhoods. To be sure, water in the Mount Airy reservoir was pumped there from the reservoir in Roxborough where some of it may have rested a bit. But at Mount Airy it would have rested a day at most when that reservoir was at capacity—and less if the water level was lower. The less full the reservoir was, the greater the chance of what was known as "direct pumpage" when river water went directly to the tap without benefit of any sedimentation, a situation which everyone sought to avoid since it presented the greatest health risk.

In Germantown direct pumpage was more or less a chronic threat, and especially troublesome because the water came from the Roxborough pumping station which was above the interceptor sewer near the city limits. In any event the city's interceptor sewer would not have helped much to keep the water safe at Roxborough because sewerage runoff in that rural section of Philadelphia was not a serious problem—the culprit was waste from the communities upstream.

In his 1883 report Ludlow had noted the danger, and nothing had changed by 1889. On the evening of 28 June residents of the area held a meeting at the hall of the Work-ingmen's Club in Germantown "to deliberate upon methods of securing a better water supply, both in quantity and quality, for that portion of the city dependent upon the Rox-borough pumping station."[21] As part of their campaign for improvements, they mailed to residents in the Germantown area a pamphlet written by a member of their committee, local physician Henry Hartshorne.

In *Our Water Supply: What It Is and What It Should be* Hartshorne said Conshohocken was not emptying its sewers in the river—but only because it had none. Norristown had nine, all flowing into the Schuylkill; Bridgeport had one, as did Pottstown, which poured into the river the "draining from 300 dwellings and several slaughterhouses and livery stables." And on up the river Hartshorne went on his sewerage survey noting more sights, like the filth-filled Man-atawny Creek, the sewer at Phoenixville, and the open drain in French Creek. "Think of it, drink of it then, if you can," he said.[22]

Hartshorne conceded that waste dumped into the Schuylkill far upstream might be rendered harmless by the flow of the river and the effects of oxygen in the air and water—this was a popular argument for doing nothing in earlier times. But the Schuylkill was not long enough or wide enough for aeration to be very effective (the Delaware per-haps was), he said, noting that the British Rivers Pollution Commission had said there was no river in Great Britain long enough "to purify itself from the noxiousness of sewage allowed to enter it."[23]

The solution that Hartshorne advocated was something new for Philadelphia: filters for the water works. As proof of their value, Hartshorne pointed to the recent research of the English chemist Percy Frankland, whose father Edward had done much of the pioneering work on developing the tests

---

[21]*Our Water Supply: The Way to Improve It: Proceedings of a Committee of Citizens of Germantown, Philadelphia* (1889), 3.
[22]Hartshorne, *Our Water Supply* . . . (1889), 17-18.
[23]Ibid., 18-19.

for water that were adopted in the 1860s. The younger Frankland tested the new filters being introduced in London, and they seemed to be very effective. Taking samples from the city's five water companies, Frankland found that the West Middlesex filter reduced the proportion of micro-organisms in each cubic centimeter of raw Thames water from 11,145 to 175; the Lambeth filter brought the same figure down to 287; Chelsea to 299; Grand Junction to 379; and Southwark to 1,526 microbes.[24] The differences in the effectiveness of the various filters, Hartshorne said, was due to a number of variables, such as the size and material of the filter, and the rate of filtration.

But the differences notwithstanding, it was obvious that filtration looked like a promising solution for Philadelphia's problems. Promising indeed, but not enough at the time to get city dollars—for reasons we will explore more fully later. The interceptor sewer and reservoirs—these were the options Philadelphians chose instead as they debated in the late 1880s and early 1890s. Given the medical and scientific uncertainties, the choices were reasonable enough and seemed to be working as the deaths from typhoid dropped steadily from a high of 785 in 1888 to 440 in 1892. To be sure, the city had stopped pumping water from the Delaware River at Kensington where the water was notoriously dirty, but this was also a sensible decision. Whatever anyone might say, Philadelphia was trying.

---

[24]Ibid., 23-24.

II. Reformers in Charge

In an age when the Democrats ruled most of the nation's large cities, Philadelphia was solidly Republican. It is not hard to see why the Grand Old Party was so popular. Philadelphia was a booming industrial center where labor and management alike would benefit from the high tariffs advocated by the GOP. The Civil War also did little for the popularity of the secessionist Democratic party. Memories of the Civil War were strong, the city having been a major hospital and supply center for the Union army. Gettysburg was also just some 120 miles from Philadelphia, bringing the fighting very close to home.

In the decades after the war the GOP worked hard to keep those memories fresh by commissioning Civil War memorials and other patriotic statuary. The influential Union League Club, founded by Republicans during the Civil War to raise troops and money, continued to work with the party, and its members believed that the American flag was more or less their exclusive property. To be sure, some Democrats won elections, but for all practical purposes Philadelphia was a one-party town by the 1890s.[1]

In the winter of 1895 a mayoral election that plays an important role in our story took place. The leading candidate for the Republican nomination was Boies Penrose, then still in the early stages of a career that would see him serve four terms in the U.S. Senate and become one of the most powerful Republicans in the state from the early 1900s to the

---

[1] For more on the Republicans and the Union League Club, see Maxwell Whitman, *Gentlemen in Crisis: The First Century of the Union League of Philadelphia, 1862-1962* (Philadelphia, 1975).

1920s. Penrose was an Old Philadelphian, in fact a Very Old Philadelphian as those things go, a scion of a family that was prominent even in colonial days. Penrose chose a career in politics a few years after his graduation from Harvard in 1880, a decision that might seem surprising given his social credentials and the generally low regard for politicians in the decades after the war because of the widespread graft in government at the time.

Public service, however, enjoyed a return to respectability in the 1880s, as elites saw themselves as the solution to the leadership problem in government. Many patrician young men were entering politics; his Harvard classmate Theodore Roosevelt, for example, also launched his own political career shortly after graduation when he won a seat in the New York state legislature in 1882. Like Roosevelt, Penrose was skillful in cultivating regulars while keeping reformers happy too, and his star rose rapidly. A state senator when he had his eye on City Hall in 1894, Penrose appeared certain to win the party's nomination—until a scandal broke shortly before the election.

Apparently someone had taken a photograph of Penrose leaving a madame's home at dawn. None of the political insiders questioned the authenticity of the photograph, the bachelor Penrose already having some notoriety along these lines, his preference for prostitutes over genteel womenfolk being one of the many ways that Penrose challenged the conventions of his own class.

Unfortunately election time was no time for any politician to allow questions to be raised about his morals, especially a candidate like Penrose who was looking for the vote of the respectable classes. Party leaders confronted Penrose with the photograph, which would appear in the papers, they said, unless he withdrew. Stunned by these last minute events, Penrose saw no choice but to drop out of the race. And so, thanks to political blackmail, a highly competent candidate lost his chance to be a mayor, a situation which was doubly unfortunate because a machine hack got the nomination and won the election, ending a period of good mayors Philadelphia had enjoyed since the late 1880s.

This is the traditional account of the election, as told many times over the years.[2] As colorful as it may be, the story does not appear to be altogether accurate. Penrose was not an overwhelmingly popular candidate, for instance, particularly in the eyes of the GOP reformers who were leery of Penrose because he was the favorite of U.S. Senator Matthew Quay, a veteran machine regular from upstate who had a notoriety of his own for graft. The reformers also already knew all about Penrose's wayward morals. Weeks before the photograph episode, they had decided to make his private life an issue, as a way of keeping him off the ticket.

The reformers organized a Committee of Ninety-Five which urged that only a candidate of spotless reputation be nominated. The committee prepared long lists of qualified candidates with Penrose's name conspicuous by its absence. Penrose ridiculed the reformers and believed he would get the nomination easily, as did most of the press.

But the Democrats were backing Robert E. Pattison, a popular patrician reformer who was completing his second term of office as governor of Pennsylvania, the only Democrat to hold that office since the Civil War. To be sure, Philadelphia had not elected a Democratic mayor since 1881—but many reform Republicans had backed Pattison as governor and Republican reformers played a critical role in 1881. Pattison might have a chance if Republicans defected again in this mayoral race, and it appeared likely they would if Penrose were nominated.

In any event, the leaders of the city GOP central committee endorsed a family man with five children who was on the lists approved by reformers. The chairman of the committee was David Martin, a powerful local boss from the nineteenth ward in blue-collar North Philadelphia. Martin was also the head of a city faction of regulars who feared that Penrose would give Quay more influence, so he had a good reason to oppose Penrose. But Martin and Quay had worked together

[2]Examples include Walter Davenport, *Power and Glory: The Life of Boies Penrose* (New York, 1931), 106-110; Robert Bowden, *Boies Penrose: A Symbol of an Era* (New York, 1937), 114-17; and more recently John Lukacs, *Philadelphia, Patricians and Philistines, 1900-1950* (New York,1981), 65; also Nathaniel Burt and Wallace E. Davies, "The Iron Age, 1876-1905" in Russell F. Weigley, ed., *Philadelphia, A 300-Year History* (New York, 1982), 497-498.

over the years, and Martin seemed to reject Penrose with considerable reluctance.

The actual selection of the candidate was left to the convention delegates, over 900 strong, who met in the Academy of Music on 9 January 1895. Furious at being snubbed by the central committee, Penrose did not drop out of the race as his biographers say he did. On the contrary Penrose campaigned harder than ever, hoping that the convention would pick him anyway. His supporters, however, were far outnumbered by the reform element and Martin regulars who united behind the central committee's choice.

As for the celebrated photograph, the first half-tone or news photograph as we know it today to appear in a mass circulation newspaper was printed in the New York *Tribune* on 21 January 1897, or more than two years later. This means that if there actually was a photograph of Penrose leaving a brothel—no print or negative is in any archive—it could not have been published on the front page of a Philadelphia newspaper in 1895. An artist's sketch could have been used (as papers illustrated stories at the time) but that certainly would not have been the same thing, so far as the credibility of the evidence was concerned.[3]

Whatever the facts about the photograph, the outcome of the 1895 mayoral election was not seen at the time as a setback for good government. Far from being a machine hack, the new mayor Charles F. Warwick, was considered a highly competent and experienced politician who had the makings of a model reform mayor like Seth Low of Brooklyn, said Rudolph Blankenburg, one of many influential GOP reformers who backed him.[4] The child of middle-class parents, Warwick was born in Philadelphia in 1850 and

---

[3]For the technical problems of using photographs in newspapers and the breakthrough in 1897, see Robert Taft, *Photography and the American Scene: A Social History, 1839-1889* (New York, 1964; orig. pub., 1938), 436-446. In 1880 a crude halftone photograph appeared in an issue of the New York *Graphic*, so technically this was the first, but the photos in papers were still in an experimental stage in those days. Taft says that printing difficulties at the time "prevented a widespread adoption of the method" (438).

[4]*Press*, 10 January 1895. Low later served a term as a reform mayor of New York after Brooklyn, Queens, the Bronx, and Staten Island joined the city in the great consolidation of 1898.

attended public schools. He clerked law in the office of a prominent attorney, E. Spenser Miller. He also took courses at the University of Pennsylvania Law School and was admitted to the bar in 1872.[5]

Interested in politics and an excellent public speaker, Warwick was soon giving talks for Republican office seekers throughout the state. He even joined the campaign team of the presidential candidate James Garfield on a trip through Ohio and Indiana in 1876. Warwick attracted the attention of the local organization in Philadelphia. He was appointed solicitor for the guardians of the poor in 1876, and in 1881 he moved up to be an assistant district attorney. Four years later he won the party's nomination for city solicitor. He put his own effective campaigning techniques to work for himself and won handily, as he did when he ran again for reelection in 1887 and 1890 and 1893.

Warwick had a reputation as an honest, hard-working, and highly competent administrator who took public service seriously. All of this augured well indeed for those who hoped to see the water crisis finally resolved during Warwick's term. The bad news about the election was the fact that many of Penrose's friends in the councils were not happy that Warwick was the new mayor. Water crisis or no, they were going to make his life unpleasant as we shall see later.

***

While the campaign was still going on, a lecture program on public health took place at the Auditorium on 14 January 1895. It was sponsored by the College of Physicians, the Wistar Institute which was affiliated with the University of Pennsylvania, the Woman's Health Protective Association, and the Civic Club. Only a handful of people showed up that bitter January evening, but two influential papers, the *Public Ledger* and the *Press*, ran lengthy stories so Philadelphians who stayed home got a chance to read about it.[6]

---

[5] Warwick biographical details from sketch in *Public Ledger*, 10 January 1895.
[6] *Public Ledger, Press*, 15 January 1896.

The main topic of interest was the research project on the Merrimac River at Lawrence, Massachusetts. Like Philadelphia, Lawrence was having problems with upstream pollution, in its case waste being carried down the river from nearby Lowell and Nashua farther up the river in neighboring New Hampshire—and from dozens of hamlets in between. Lawrence had a typhoid rate four times the average in Massachusetts in the early 1890s, and worse even than Philadelphia's at the time.

In 1887 the Massachusetts state board of health had established a laboratory called the "experimental station," where scientists were studying water pollution at Lawrence. Recognized as the leading research center on pollution in the country, the laboratory attracted many academics because few colleges and universities at the time had such good research facilities. William Thompson Sedwick, for example, a biologist at the Massachusetts Institute of Technology, worked with students at the lab in developing new standards of water testing that were accepted by the state in 1890.[7]

The most important news from Lawrence was that the typhoid rate had dropped dramatically since 1893, thanks to the filter the scientists had designed. Water was pumped from the Merrimac River to a reservoir and then filtered through a bed of fine sand at the bottom. Between two and two and one-half million gallons were being filtered this way daily at Lawrence, and similar filters with larger capacities could easily be built in Philadelphia.

The speaker on the filters was T.W. Drown, a chemist and another M.I.T. researcher at the lab. The relationship between the filter and the decline of typhoid was simply "a statement of cause and effect," he said. A native of Philadelphia, Drown also told his audience that he had defended the city for years against insinuations of slowness, but he could no longer justify her procrastination in light of the Lawrence results. Philadelphia has three options, he said:

1st. To remove the source of pollution.
2nd. To abandon the supply and get a better one.

[7]Barbara G. Rosenkrantz, *Public Health and the State: Changing Views in Massachusetts, 1842-1936* (Cambridge, Mass., 1972), 99-102.

3rd. To purify the water by sand filtration.

"Whether it is possible in the case of Philadelphia to do either the first or the second I leave to competent and disinterested engineers," he added, but he felt that "Philadelphia can get perfectly safe drinking water from the Schuylkill in its present condition by constructing a sand filter as Lawrence has done."[8] To be sure, filters were not unknown to Philadelphians. As we saw earlier, a pamphlet on filters had been distributed to Germantowners in 1889.

And there had been interest in filters in 1892 when dreaded cholera threatened Europe and America. Cholera—a cousin of typhoid but more feared and frightening because it was so virulent—established itself in the intestines. Rapid dehydration followed, caused by violent vomiting and diarrhea. Death could occur within days, sometimes hours. An Edinburgh surgeon who had seen cholera victims in India described the symptoms:[9]

The eyes surrounded by a dark circle are completely sunken into the sockets, the whole countenance is collapsed, the skin livid. . . . The surface [of the skin] is now generally covered with cold sweat, the nails are blue, and the skin of the hands and feet are corrugated as if they had been long steeped in water. . . . The voice is hollow and unnatural. If the case be accompanied by spasms, the suffering of the patient is much aggravated, and is sometimes excruciating. . . .

As William H. McNeill has noted, the Western powers, and Great Britain in particular, broke the regional and cultural barriers that had long contained the disease in the East. Taking control of India in the eighteenth century, British colonial armies moved freely around the subcontinent and helped to "stir up the great well of infection."[10]

The death tolls were high when the first epidemic struck in the West in the late 1820s and early 1830s. Some 30,000 were estimated to have died in Great Britain and 20,000 in the United States. Philadelphia was among the cities struck,

---

[8]*Press*, 15 January 1896.
[9]R.J. Morris, *Cholera 1832* (London, 1976), 16. Like typhoid, cholera is still a potential threat, but vaccines also control it.
[10]McNeill, *Plagues and People* (Garden City, 1976), 230ff. Other useful references are Charles E. Rosenberg, *The Cholera Years* (Chicago, 1962); Roderick E. McGrew, *Russia and the Cholera, 1823-1832* (Madison, Wis., 1965).

but fortunately not as hard as New York—thanks in large part to the Fairmount water works which provided safe enough water in the first half of the century at least, and plenty of water for street cleaning as well. New Yorkers noted the lower disease rate in Philadelphia and a team of officials came to inspect the Fairmount works in the fall of 1832. Impressed, they went home and began pushing for the water reform that resulted in the Croton aqueduct.[11] Fortunately basic improvements in sanitation like interceptor sewers and Croton water could make a difference, and cholera was no longer much of a threat after the 1860s in America or western Europe.

But cholera remained a headache in Russia and other less progressive countries in eastern Europe. It could strike again from there—and this is what happened in 1892. Most likely carried by immigrants from Russia, cholera was reported in several cities including the port of Hamburg where a major epidemic occurred. Philadelphians understandably worried since ships could carry the disease across the Atlantic.

As part of an international effort to check cholera, the president of the United States on 1 September 1892 ordered all ships sailing from Europe with immigrants aboard, leaving that day or after, to remain in quarantine for at least twenty days when they arrived in America. Although not required, the Philadelphia board of health also had all the steerage passengers take baths.

The quarantine hospital on the Delaware in Tinicum Township south of Philadelphia did not have adequate facilities to handle large numbers, so the board decided to lease and outfit a steamer familiar to many Philadelphians: the *Georgeanna*, an old daytrip excursion boat that plied the Schuylkill above Fairmount in the summertime. Twenty-four bath tubs were put on board, in separate rooms for men and women. Their clothing was also sanitized in a large box-like container that produced a steam spray of 220 degrees fahrenheit. Cholera was a hardy microbe, but it could not survive temperatures that high.[12]

---

[11]Nelson M. Blake, *Water*, 133ff.
[12]Board of Health, *Annual Report* (1892), 29ff. Even though it was outside Phila-

The first ship from Europe to arrive in Philadelphia after the presidential order was the *Ohio* with 646 passengers aboard. The *Ohio* having sailed from Liverpool on 31 August, the quarantine requirement did not apply. But before crossing the ocean, the *Ohio* made a stop at Queensland (Cobh) in Ireland where it picked up twenty-four Irish immigrants. This gave it a "mixed" passenger list, which meant the ship might have to stay the full twenty days. The cabin class passengers in particular were upset at that prospect. The ship had been fumigated in Liverpool before sailing, and no one took ill during the ocean journey. In any event, after sitting out six days at anchor in the Delaware River and having steerage passengers and their belongings go through the *Georgeanna*, the *Ohio* was allowed to dock in Philadelphia on 16 September.[13] By the end of October another nineteen ships came, for a total of 1,907 passengers and crew. Many of the ships were freighters carrying only a few passengers (the *Pennsylvania* with 559 passengers was the only other large ship). They went through the same routine as the *Ohio*.

To be sure, the washing and steam spray may have been an indignity to some, but they were inspired by understandable concerns about contagion. Health officials worried that some of the passengers in steerage—many of them immigrants— might have carried cholera from eastern Europe, or come into contact with it in their travels westward. (On the *Ohio* most of the immigrants were from the British Isles and Scandinavia, but some were from Germany and Poland and other countries in eastern and southern Europe.) Health officials also worried about contagion among the steerage passengers.

Steerage was cheap travel space for the working classes, and few immigrants could afford to pay more. In earlier times an ocean journey in steerage was an ordeal not every-

delphia, the quarantine hospital (called the Lazaretto) was run for years by the city board of health. In 1893 the state took over. The hospital was closed two years later when it appeared to be no longer needed. Apparently after 1895 shipboard ill were taken to the city's municipal hospital as they frequently were before when the Lazaretto was not open (usually fall and winter). See Edward T. Mormon, "Guarding Against Alien Impurities: The Philadelphia Lazaretto, 1854-1893," *Pennsylvania Magazine of History and Biography* 108 (April 1984), 131-151.

[13]Some of the passengers were so annoyed with the delay that they presented a formal protest to the board of health. *Inquirer,* 17 Sept. 1982.

one survived, but by the late nineteenth century, ships were healthier places and steerage was more like "super economy" today. To be sure, accommodations varied greatly among ships—in some, steerage included a bunk in a small crowded cabin; others, with rows of wooden benches, looked like waiting rooms in a train station. (Steerage passengers on the *Ohio* had beds and cabins—the ship must have been heavily involved in immigrant travel because 405 of its passengers were in that class.) In some of the ships that catered to the affluent classes, the steerage passengers were confined to areas below decks. This helped to contain disease, but it did not keep steerage passengers healthy. In any event, it was fears about cholera that inspired the cleaning measures—not nativism since the washing and spraying did not apply to an immigrant in the cabin classes. (Crews also bathed, and their quarters were sprayed.)

The only one real scare in the United States came in New York, which was the main port of entry for immigrants from Europe—and where most of the ships from cholera-stricken Hamburg headed. Several deaths were reported in September, but the board of health acted quickly to prevent a serious outbreak. Nobody became ill in Philadelphia. Dr. D.W. Thompson, the physician in charge of the *Georgeanna*, praised "the wise foresight" of the board of health, whose action had successfully protected Philadelphia's "million of people and its billion of capital, both of which were in serious danger and would have suffered incalculable loss had a single case of imported cholera appeared at the wharves of the city."[14] Considering that New York had a few cases and survived, Thompson's remarks were an exaggeration, but they suggest the anxiety at the time.

As for cholera and filtration, with the outbreak in Europe already in the news, the Philadelphia city councils in June of 1892 approved an ordinance to build an experimental filtration station on the Schuylkill. When the threat passed, however, the councils never allocated any money. In 1893 a depression began which also discouraged spending on experimental projects. The water bureau complained, but it

---

[14]Board of Health, *Annual Report* (1892), 37.

did not complain very loudly, however, given the economy, and the dollars the bureau was getting for more reservoirs to increase sedimentation. In any case, by 1895 the depression was over, and filtration had proven itself in the United States at Lawrence. As Drown said, Philadelphia now had an example it could emulate.

***

Another promising development during this period was the widespread acceptance, at long last, of germ theory within the medical profession. To be sure, some still clung to their miasmist views, but they were now clearly in the minority, given the overwhelming evidence of the breakthroughs in bacteriology. In October of 1894, a committee of the board of health chaired by Dr. William H. Ford recommended that the board establish a bacteriological division within the health department. New York had already done this in 1892, under the leadership of a distinguished public health physician, Dr. Herman Biggs, and the committee felt this was an example worth emulating. The board adopted the report, and the city councils promptly funded the full request for $15,000 for a bacteriologist, support staff, and laboratory expenses.[15]

To help get the lab underway, the University of Pennsylvania offered several rooms free of rent in its Laboratory of Hygiene. The provost of the University at the time was William Pepper, a highly regarded Philadelphia physician and educator who was keenly interested in public health and the water issue in particular. (Pepper would have chaired the meeting at which Drown spoke had he not been called to Washington on other business.) The lab would be an independent facility which the board of health would run in conformity with its own rules and regulations, the university said in its offer.

The only stipulation the university made was that the chief

---

[15]Board of Health, *Annual Report* (1894), 138-139.

of the lab be selected from the staff at the Laboratory of Hygiene, a request that did not seem unreasonable since the Penn lab was a highly regarded research center. However attractive the offer may have been in some ways, the city decided to put the new lab in City Hall where the chemistry lab and other health department offices were located. It opened officially on 10 May 1895.

For the staff in the new division of bacteriology, typhoid of course was just one of many diseases that they sought to study and control, diphtheria, scarlet fever, smallpox, German measles, meningitis, and tuberculosis being among the other serious problems at the time. In fact typhoid was one of the diseases they could do least about in a direct way to prevent since no antitoxins had been developed yet as they had been for smallpox and diphtheria. (A typhoid vaccine would be in wide use by World War I.)

Even more frustrating for health department officials, typhoid was then considered one of the "preventable diseases" in the sense that the major cause was known by then to be polluted water. In reviewing mortality statistics for 1896, the head of the department noted that the typhoid deaths for the year had dropped to 402, down 67 from the previous year, and with the exception of 1894 the 1896 figure was the lowest since 1879. Even so, he said, these were 402 needless deaths because preventive measures could exclude "this disease from the mortuary records." With almost an audible sigh, he concluded by remarking that "In the report last year reference is made to the prevailing causes of typhoid fever in this city, and therefore it is unnecessary to go over the subject again."[16]

The water bureau was the city department that could do something. It was under the leadership of John C. Trautwine, Jr., a respected civil engineer in his 40s whom Warwick had appointed chief in 1895. The son of a prominent Philadelphia civil engineer and architect, Trautwine attended public schools and then studied engineering under his father and assisted him in revising the popular *Civil Engineer's Handbook* and other engineering works that his father had

---

[16]Ibid. (1896), 36-37.

written.[17] The younger Trautwine worked for many years
with Morris, Wheeler & Co., a iron and steel manufacturer
in Philadelphia. When his father died in 1883, Trautwine
left the firm and took over his father's consulting practice
and continued to edit and revise his father's works, which
remained popular.

Trautwine served as an unpaid "dollar a year" engineer in
the water bureau for several years in the 1880s and then left
in 1889 for two years of study in Great Britain and Europe.
On his return to Philadelphia, Trautwine remained as busy
as ever in professional affairs, serving as secretary of the
American Society of Civil Engineers and business manager
and editor of its weekly journal; as director of the Engineers
Club and a member of the board of managers of the Franklin
Institute, which until recently was a center for research in
science and technology as well as a museum. (As of 1984, the
museum and research center became separate and independent operations.) Vigorous and younger looking than his
years, with a short haircut and a neatly trimmed beard,
Trautwine could be brusque and outspoken, but his pep and
professionalism seemed to be just what the water bureau
needed.

The "first and most pressing duty" of his bureau was to
curtail "the reckless waste of water," Trautwine said in his
first annual report.[18] Water waste indeed. What about the
typhoid crisis? Actually the two were interrelated as he saw
the problem. Despite the increase in reservoir capacity in
recent years, consumption was climbing faster, which meant
in effect that the sedimentation or "resting" process could
not be expected to protect the city's water supply. This would
be bad enough, but Trautwine believed that a good deal of
the consumption was not consumption at all but simply waste
caused by careless consumers.

To support his case, Trautwine cited the results of a bureau investigation in 1895 of water consumption in 142 new
houses in a neighborhood in North Philadelphia. There

[17]Trautwine biographical details from sketch in *Public Ledger*, 11 November 1899;
also *Who's Who in America,1897-1942*, 1: 1251. Some information on his father as
architect is in James F. O'Gorman et al., *Drawing Toward Building: Philadelphia Archi-
tectural Graphics, 1732-1986* (Philadelphia, 1986), 74-75.
[18]Bureau of Water, *Annual Report* (1895), 99.

were a total of 782 faucets, flush toilets, and sundry other water devices in the seven-room houses, of which 22 leaked slightly and 32 were running continuously. Consumption for a twenty-four hour period was 119,800 gallons, of which 103,680 was considered wasted. Using per capita figures and given 539 residents in the houses, the bureau figured that of the 222 gallons that were pumped for each person, only 30 gallons were actually used, the rest going from the tap down the drain.

The findings were especially disturbing because an estimated 90 percent of the city's water was consumed in homes.[19] Trautwine believed the money wasted pumping unused water could go toward building filtration plants. He was abreast of all the recent developments, and he wanted to see filtration implemented in Philadelphia. It would be expensive but less so if the city eliminated waste and filtered only the water it was using.

Trautwine wanted an ordinance requiring water meters in all homes and businesses. Noting that an ordinance for the voluntary metering ordinance of businesses had been in effect since 1872, Trautwine said his proposal was simply extending the scope of an existing law and making it mandatory. He noted also that previous water bureau chiefs including Ludlow had made similar recommendations so his idea was not novel. The purpose, he assured everyone, was not to increase revenue but rather "to decrease the city's expenditure by cutting off a waste, which under present circumstances appeared little short of criminal." The amount of water allowed with the set fee would be more than adequate for normal household use so "nothing could be gained by economizing," lest anyone worry that meters would restrict unduly the use of water "particularly on the part of the poorer members of our population."

The proposed ordinance would simply cover the city's costs to provide home service, he said. Manufacturers' rates could even be set below cost if this would mollify opposition to mandatory metering for everyone.[20] Far from being the enemy of the people, the water bureau and its parent, the

---

[19]Ibid.
[20]Ibid., 98.

department of public works, were in Trautwine's words, "a socialistic or communistic organization, by means of which the entire community seeks to obtain certain results to the best advantage and at a reasonable cost."[21]

Unfortunately for Trautwine, Philadelphians were not interested in mandatory meters. Indeed the citizenry had begun to view the unlimited usage of water as something akin to a God-given right which few councilmen cared to challenge in the 1890s or for years after that—Philadelphia did not adopt a mandatory meter system until 1919 and it was one of the last major cities to do so.

Trautwine met less resistance when he introduced his other major proposal, a request for $250,000 to build an experimental filtration station where different kinds of filters could be tested—in effect the proposal that the councils adopted during the cholera scare of 1892 but never funded. Louisville, Kentucky, was building an experimental station, he told the councilmen, and this approach would be a good way to make sure that Philadelphia picked the proper filters for its own water conditions.[22] Trautwine also noted that the station could filter the entire water supply of a small district, like the one served by Belmont in West Philadelphia, so the station would have immediate practical value.

As for the filters, the ones most widely used at the time were called slow sand filters, like the one at Lawrence. Raw water was first pumped into a sedimentation basin to "rest" awhile. Then it went to the filter beds and percolated through several feet of sand before going to a holding reservoir or in some cases directly into the distributing mains. Bacteria, of course, were smaller than the finest grains of sand. In theory they should have been able to pass through such filters however deep the sand. But a jelly-like film of bacteria formed on the upper layer of sand, and this kept nearly all the rest of the bacteria from getting through, a phenomenon German scientists called a "Schultsdeck" or "dirt cover." A single foot of sand could act as an effective filter if it were properly coated. A deeper bed of four or five feet, however, was considered better because even more bac-

---

[21]Ibid.
[22]Ibid., 127-128.

teria got caught along the way—and a deeper bed was safer, should the dirt cover on the top be accidentally broken.[23]

The other filter choice was the "rapid" or "mechanical" type. They were usually circular tanks, around ten feet wide and four feet deep, with a sand filter two to three feet deep at the bottom and pipes underneath to carry the filtered water off to a reservoir. The rapid sand filters worked on the principle of a mixing vat. As raw water was pumped into the tank, a chemical solution usually of aluminum sulfate was added. It quickly coagulated and coated the top of the filter with a jelly-like substance similar to the natural bacteria dirt cover of the slow sand filter. As their name implies, rapid filters had high rates of filtration which meant that more water could be filtered this way.

Given the greater filtering rate, the obvious choice would seem to be the rapid filter, but city officials had to consider a variety of factors. The rapid filters, for example, had a greater element of risk since they depended on the careful addition of coagulants to create an effective dirt cover. Slow filters on the other hand did not work as well as rapid filters in cleaning up a muddy river—which the Schuylkill often was when freshets surged down the valley. Choosing the right kind for the city's needs was a tricky business made even trickier because water filters in the 1890s were much like the microcomputers of the 1980s: a new field where the technology was in the midst of rapid change.

In any event, the joint finance and water committees approved the ordinance for the experimental stations by wide majorities with little fuss. But the bill was clearly in trouble on 5 March 1896 when Thomas Meehan from Germantown challenged it.

Meehan was an uncommon councilman. Born in England in 1826 and the son of a gardener, he studied horticulture at the Royal Botanic Gardens at Kew near London before coming to Philadelphia in 1848. He worked at Robert Buist's nurseries and on the estate of Caleb Cope in Holmesburg before starting his own nursery business in 1852 in German-

---

[23]References on the filters include James H. Fuertes, *Water Filtration Works* (New York, 1907); and Milton Stein, *Water Purification Plants and their Operations* (New York, 1926, 3rd ed.).

town with William Saunders. Meehan was soon sole owner and his firm prospered, earning for itself a reputation as one of the best in the country for its trees and shrubs. Meehan edited the *Gardener's Monthly* and after that his own *Meehan's Monthly* subtitled "A Magazine of Horticulture, Botany and kindred subjects." He was also an author of several books including *The American Handbook of Ornamental Trees* (1853) and *Native Flowers and Ferns of the United States* (two volumes, 1878-79), which established his reputation as a scholar in the fields of horticulture and botany.[24]

In addition to all this, Meehan was keenly interested in civic affairs. In his 60s he turned over much of the nursery business to his sons and went into the common council as member of the 22nd ward delegation representing Germantown. With a dozen years of service by 1896, Meehan was considered an elder statesman—and he looked like one, with his snowy hair and beard.

Meehan was a man of strong opinions especially in water matters. For starters, he opposed Trautwine's water bill because the experimental station would assist only a small fraction of the city's residents. If any filtering were to be done, it should be from a large reservoir north of the city that would benefit everyone. But filtration really made no sense, Meehan said, because many bacteria were recognized as harmless and might even be beneficial. Dangerous microorganisms seemed to get through the best of filters anyway. During the 1892 cholera epidemic in Europe, a serious outbreak occurred in the German city of Altona near Hamburg, he said, despite the presence of a filter. In sum, filters did not work, and the current policy of sedimentation was sound.

After Meehan finished, a number of other councilmen argued along the same lines, the most outspoken being William R. Knight, Jr., a machine regular from the 25th ward in Kensington who declared that the advice of engineers and scientists was "all bosh." He said "It was time for councilmen to rely on their own common sense." On went the opponents of the filtration, talking so long in fact that no vote could be taken that day.[25]

---

[24]Biographical information from Meehan file in Germantown Historical Society.
[25]*Press*, 6 March 1896.

At the request of the head of the department of public works, Thomas M. Thompson, Trautwine prepared a written reply that appeared in many of the papers. He strongly differed with Meehan and his colleagues. Sedimentation was simply no longer safe enough, he said, given the vastly more effective protection filters provided. Trautwine included charts and tables of data from other cities that showed the benefit of filtration over sedimentation. The city, however, could not rely on the experience of others, given all the different operating conditions. An experimental station that would serve a portion of the city was the best way to proceed before investing "larger sums."

Trautwine went on to challenge Meehan's views on bacteria. "Mr. Meehan would hardly claim that any bacteria are so beneficial as to justify us in seeking contaminated water or even in neglecting means for its purification," he commented. Trautwine felt it wiser to consider all bacteria as a potential threat, like "bullets in battle," and if filters could cut that threat down to one or two percent, it certainly made sense to do so. As for Meehan's remarks about Altona, Trautwine quoted from the same source to show that the cholera had swept the city only after severe cold weather had frozen the filters and temporarily put them out of operation.

Far from being ineffective, the filters had given Altona a death rate of only 221 per 100,000 in that epidemic compared to 1,350 per 100,000 in neighboring Hamburg which did not have a filter at that time. Along a street that marked the dividing line between the two cities, houses on the Hamburg side were "rampant" with cholera, he said, while on the Altona side "not one case occurred," striking evidence indeed that filtration made a difference.[26]

Trautwine's reply seemed convincing to the members of the Engineers Club, which was one of the many groups that endorsed the filtration project. Referring to the work going on for a sanitary canal that would take sewerage away from Lake Michigan, one member said, "If Chicago can afford to spend $17 million for the disposal of its sewerage, surely we can afford to appropriate a quarter of a million dollars for

---

[26]*Press*, 10 March 1896.

this first step in the permanent improvement of the water supply."[27]

The Woman's Health Protective Association sent every councilman a letter urging him to vote favorably on the ordinance since "science has demonstrated everywhere that filtration will remove disease germs and dirt from polluted water."[28] T.M. Drown, the scientist at the Lawrence lab who was now president of Lehigh University, also lobbied for the bill. In an open letter to the head of the department of public works, Drown said, "It is inconceivable that with the indisputable facts before them, there should be any members of the councils who hesitate to provide means to filter the Schuylkill water that it may be both clear and wholesome."[29]

Despite the public persuasion during the week, Meehan and his friends did not change their minds. When the common council met again on 12 March, once again they said the same things and kept up the filibustering so no vote was taken that day either. Meehan, who had the floor when the meeting ended, took up where he left off when they convened again on March 19.

Whatever the scientific experts may say about the benefits of filtration, Meehan still believed that sedimentation was good enough. Shall we take up a costly policy of filtration which will take decades to complete, he asked, "or spend $250,000 to mend our leaky reservoirs which will give us water like this," as he held up a bottle of clear water he said came from a reservoir after two days of subsidence.[30] "Public opinion has been manufactured in favor of this bill," he said. "The mere fact that there is a majority against us should not influence us," Meehan told his friends in the council. "If majorities had counted, the world would be barbarianism today. The Master himself when he was on earth was in the minority, but we concede that the majority were wrong."[31]

Wearying of Meehan's rhetoric, Edward A. Anderson, the speaker of the council, said he was surprised that a gen-

[27]*Public Ledger*, 19 March 1896.
[28]*Press*, 11 March 1896.
[29]*Press*, 10 March 1896.
[30]*Public Ledger*, 20 March 1896.
[31]Ibid.

tleman as educated as Meehan could still believe in subsidence as a remedy. Eight years ago, Anderson said, he had heard Meehan make the same argument to support the building of the East Park reservoir, but the water was just as bad now as it was then. Knight and others behind Meehan quickly came to his defense and continued the filibustering.

The supporters of the filtration were finally able to force a vote that day. The majority of the members of the common council voted yes, 49-37, but they were unable to get the two-thirds majority necessary for appropriation bills. So the measure was dead, and it never even came up for a vote in the select council.

It is impossible, of course, to say exactly why the vote went the way it did. Factional infighting no doubt had something to do with it, the bill having been proposed by Trautwine who was appointed by Warwick, who in turn was not admired by Penrose supporters in the councils, many of whom did in fact vote against the measure.

As for Meehan, he was not a Penrose man, so in his case at least that explanation seems less likely. He certainly outraged the editor of the *Germantown Telegraph* and other Germantowners who were fighting hard for filtration. Shortly afterward, under the leadership of businessman Frank J. Firth, Germantowners organized the City Organizations' Filtration Committee as a city-wide consortium to push for a filtration ordinance—and Meehan clearly inspired their decision. Like many others, the *Press* was baffled and bitter. It commented that[32]

The people of Philadelphia owe a good deal to Mr. Thomas Meehan and respect him. He has been the persistent advocate and promoter of a liberal and widely extended system of small parks. Almost alone among Councilmen he has shown an intelligent interest in the subject of street shade trees. He knows what they should be and what is their value. If his efforts could have accomplished it, we would before this have had a fish hatchery on the banks of the Schuylkill east of the Zoological Garden. When a city forester was to be selected, everyone recognized the fitness of Mr. Thomas Meehan's appointment as one of the commissioners to

---

[32]*Press*, 27 March 1896. Clipping in scrapbook in papers of Frank J. Firth, Germantown Historical Society.

examine the applications and recommend a fit person for city forester and gardener.

It was to be presumed, therefore, judging from his usual liberal and progressive spirit, that Mr. Meehan would be found leading the ranks of the filtrationists. This the more because he comes from Germantown, that wealthy and enlightened suburb of Philadelphia, which labors under the disadvantage of having the worst water of any portion of the city. . . . It is amazing, therefore, that an intelligent Germantown Councilman should be found leading the forces of reaction, prejudice and ignorance against filtration. . . . We welcome the statement that Mr. Meehan believes filtration would be a benefit to the entire city and that he only opposes it because of the supposed long wait for its benefit that some sections would have to endure. Let him lead a crusade for filtration for the entire city and readjust his time estimate by consulting competent engineers. Then will the Germantown Councilman be again worthy of his reputation and be withdrawn from his alliance with mossbacks, the uninstructed and the uninstructible, who assisted him in killing the $250,000 appropriation for making a start toward the filtration of the city's water.

In fairness to Meehan, he seemed hard put to accept the germ theory, given his Unitarian faith in a rational world. In his preface to the bound annual volume of his *Meehan's Monthly* for 1896, he says

All nature is a series of advances and rests. We work by day and sleep by night. Plants and flowers have no diurnal periods—but they rest and advance all the same. Their whole growth is in rhythms. A little movement—a greater swell—a gentle passage to rest. Then comes a renewal, many times daily with its corresponding rest.

Meehan loved Mother Nature—and he seemed to doubt that she would create something so evil as invisible microbes that killed people. Many others still doubted too, the most noteworthy at the time being the German doctor who in 1892 swallowed a beaker of water filled with cholera microbes to "disprove" the germ theory. The good doctor suffered no harm, no doubt because stomach acids managed to kill all the germs. The fact, however, that he was willing to take such risks was an indication that old beliefs did not change overnight.[33]

---

[33]McNeill, *Plagues and People*, 236.

Notwithstanding his philosophical views, it should be noted that Meehan had other possible motives for opposing the bill. He was a politician who liked to deliver for his constituents, and he was understandably cool to an experimental filtration in West Philadelphia that would not directly benefit his ward in Germantown.

In any event, Trautwine did not help his cause any by his handling of Meehan—who was blustery and opinionated, to be sure, but a distinguished citizen nonetheless and someone who required delicate treatment. Showing the councilman up in print was an impolitic move, and after that Meehan seemed to go after Trautwine and his bill with extra zeal.

Trautwine may have made another tactical error in seeking only limited funding. To critics of filtration, this could have been read as a sign that Trautwine himself was not sure enough to ask for the full amount necessary. Some of the councilmen may have been unwilling to support a project that seemed intimidating even to Trautwine, who emphasized all the complicated variables. In his written reply to council critics, for example, he said[34]

We are required to determine not only which is, on general principles, the best of several systems of filtration in use; not only which would be the best for the waters with which we have to deal (for what is best for one is by no means necessarily the best for another), but also what sort and arrangement of plan is best adapted to the requirements of each of the several localities at which our filters would have to be erected, to what extent we must provide for sedimentation of the water before filtration, how that sedimentation can be best and most economically effected, and many other matters which cannot be learned from the experience of other communities operating under conditions different from our own, but only from experience upon the conditions obtaining here. It is most important that we should have this information before proceeding to the investment of larger sums.

Whatever the reasons for the opposing votes, a majority of the councilmen had supported filtration. Even more encouraging was the remark of Councilman Knight, who said he voted against the bill because there was no need for experi-

---

[34]*Press*, 10 March 1896.

mentation. The water bureau should propose instead a city-wide plan. "Let someone show me where to get that amount of money, and I will cheerfully vote for an appropriation."[35]

A bond issue was seen as the solution, and in November the common council approved an ordinance for a loan by a vote of 99-3, with Thomas Meehan—still opposed—among the three.[36] In December the select council also backed the idea by a nearly unanimous 33-1 vote. In March Drown had asked, "How long will patient Philadelphia have the reproach of drinking foul water and willfully sacrificing hundreds of lives each year?"[37] As 1896 ended, it looked like the waiting was over.

---

[35]Ibid., 20 March 1896.
[36]When threatened with a ward revolt the next year, Meehan pledged to support filtration. He was still representing Germantown (and voting for filtration) when he died on 19 November 1901 at the age of seventy-five. For the dispute in 1897, see 6 January editorial in *Germantown Telegraph* and related clippings in Firth scrapbook.
[37]Ibid., 19 March 1896.

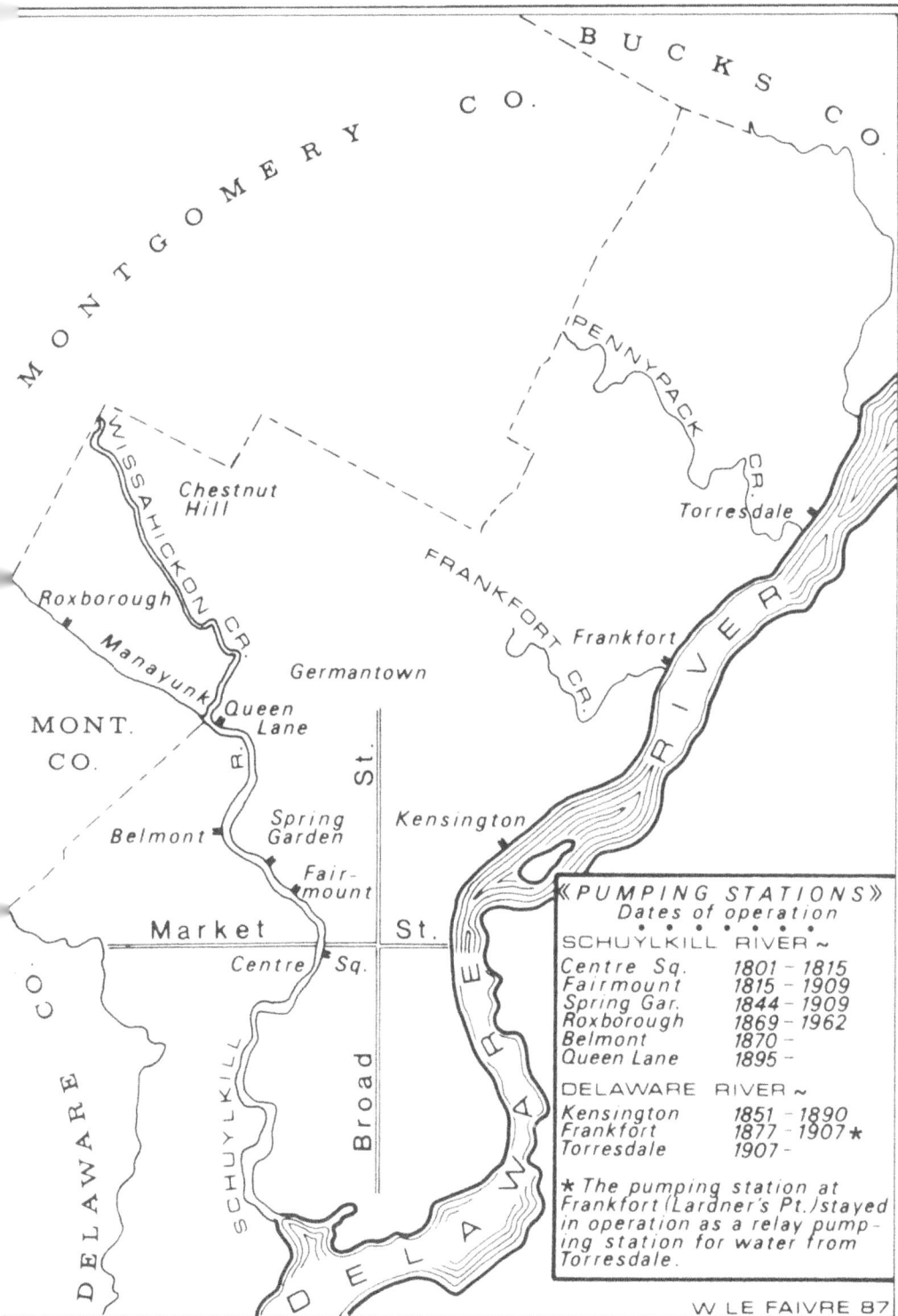

B U C K S   C O.

M O N T G O M E R Y   C O.

PENNYPACK CR.

WISSAHICKON CR.

Chestnut
Hill

Torresdale

Roxborough

FRANKFORT CR.

Frankfort

Manayunk

Germantown

Queen
Lane

MONT.
CO.

R.

St.

Kensington

Belmont

Spring
Garden

Fair-
mount

R I V E R

Market   St.

Centre   Sq.

Broad

SCHUYLKILL

D E L A W A R E

DELAWARE CO.

《 P U M P I N G   S T A T I O N S 》
Dates of operation
· · · · · · ·
SCHUYLKILL   RIVER ~

Centre Sq.	1801 – 1815
Fairmount	1815 – 1909
Spring Gar.	1844 – 1909
Roxborough	1869 – 1962
Belmont	1870 –
Queen Lane	1895 –

DELAWARE   RIVER ~

Kensington	1851 – 1890
Frankfort	1877 – 1907 *
Torresdale	1907 –

* The pumping station at
Frankfort (Lardner's Pt.) stayed
in operation as a relay pumping station for water from
Torresdale.

W LE FAIVRE 87

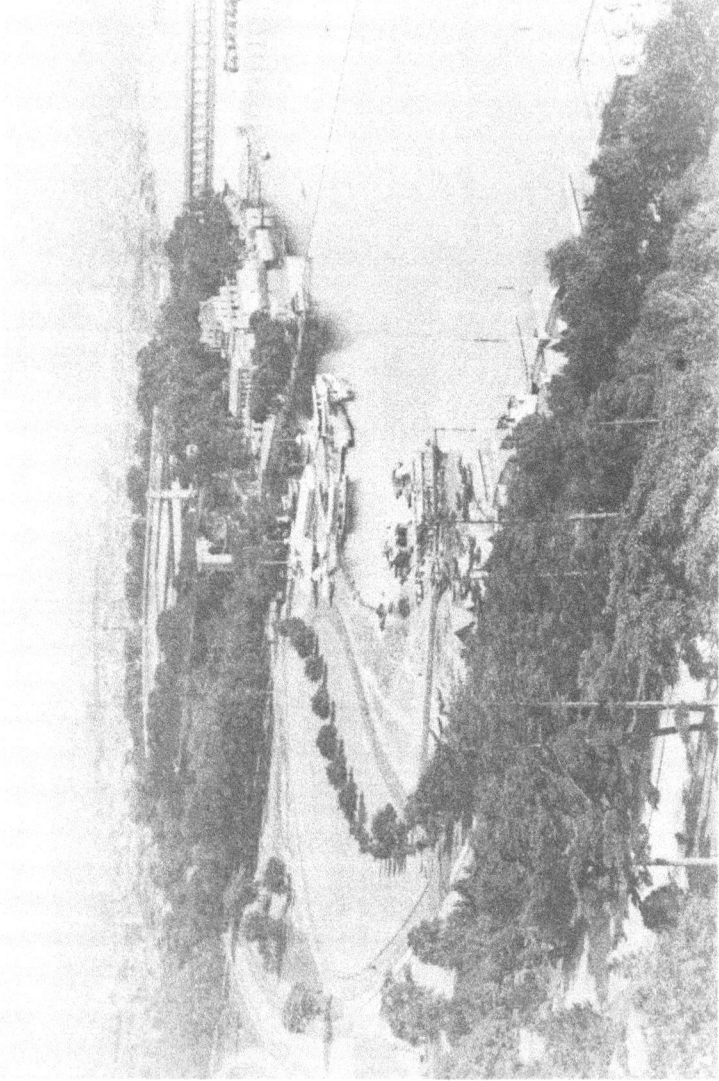

Fairmount water works in 1876. Reservoir atop Fairmount had a capacity of 26.3 million gallons. The works served neighborhoods in center city and south Philadelphia. Courtesy of the Free Library.

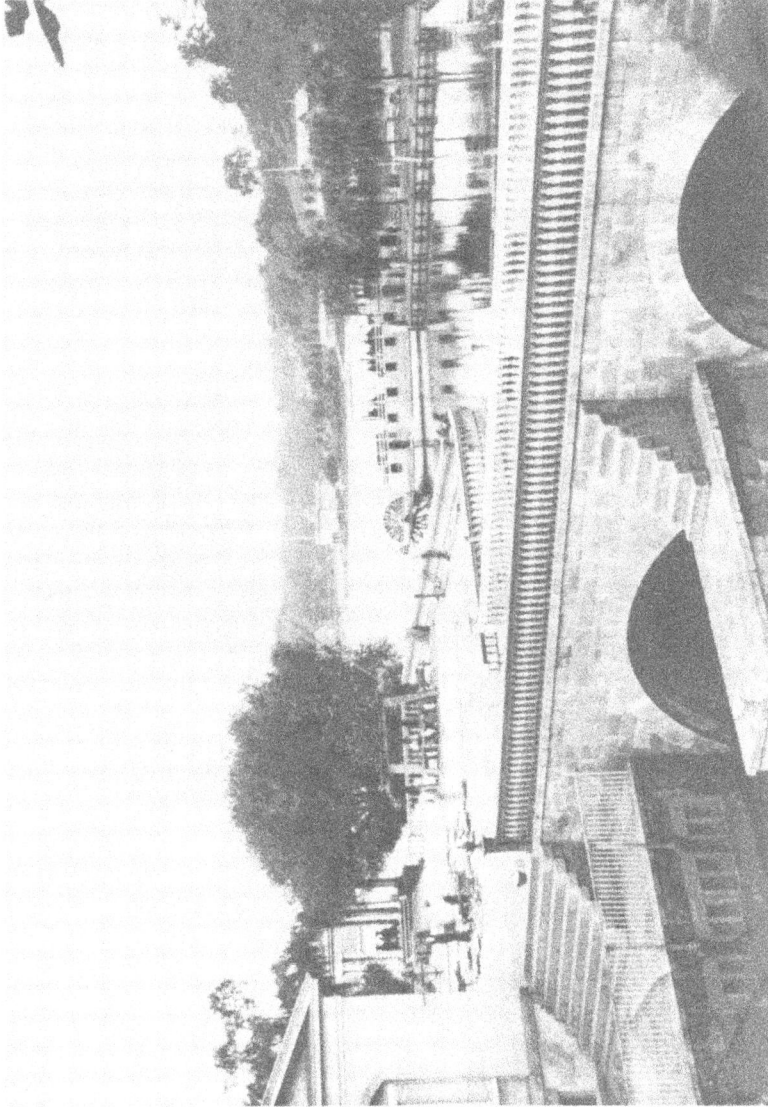

Forebay of Fairmount water works around 1870. The paddle-wheeler was one of the many day boats that plied the Schuylkill above the dam. (The dock was across from the forebay.) Boat House Row is in the background. Courtesy of the Free Library.

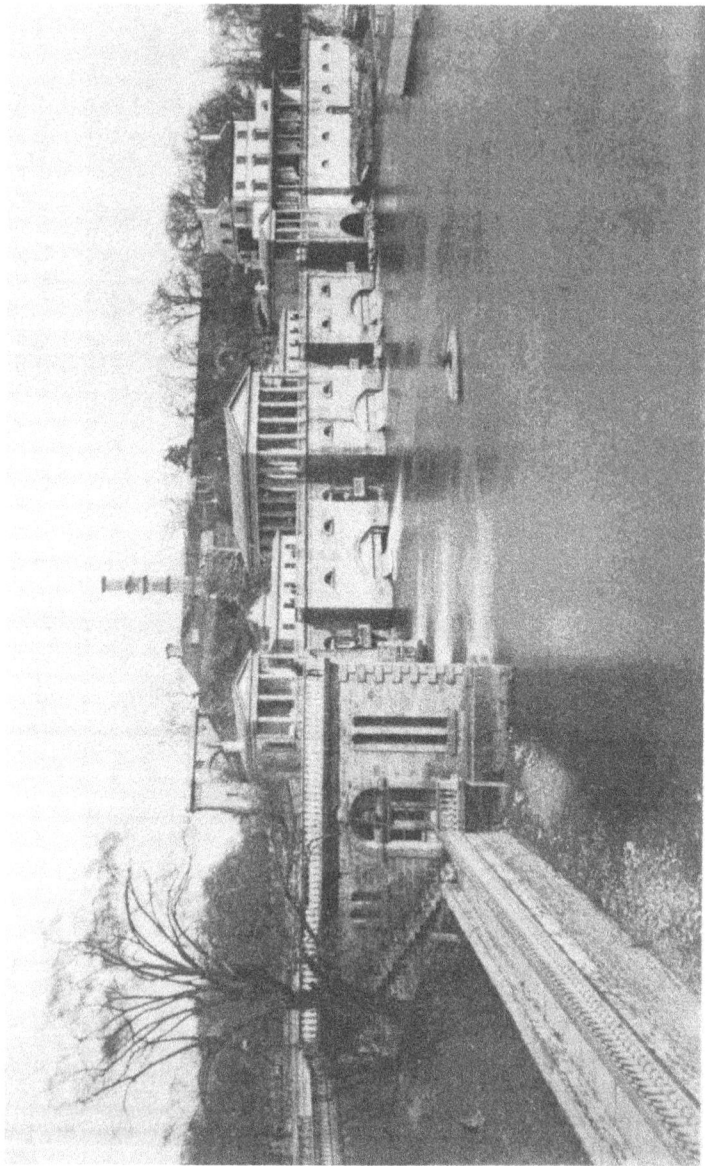

Fairmount water works in the 1890s. The campanile-like tower is a standpipe that increased water pressure. Courtesy of Germantown Historical Society.

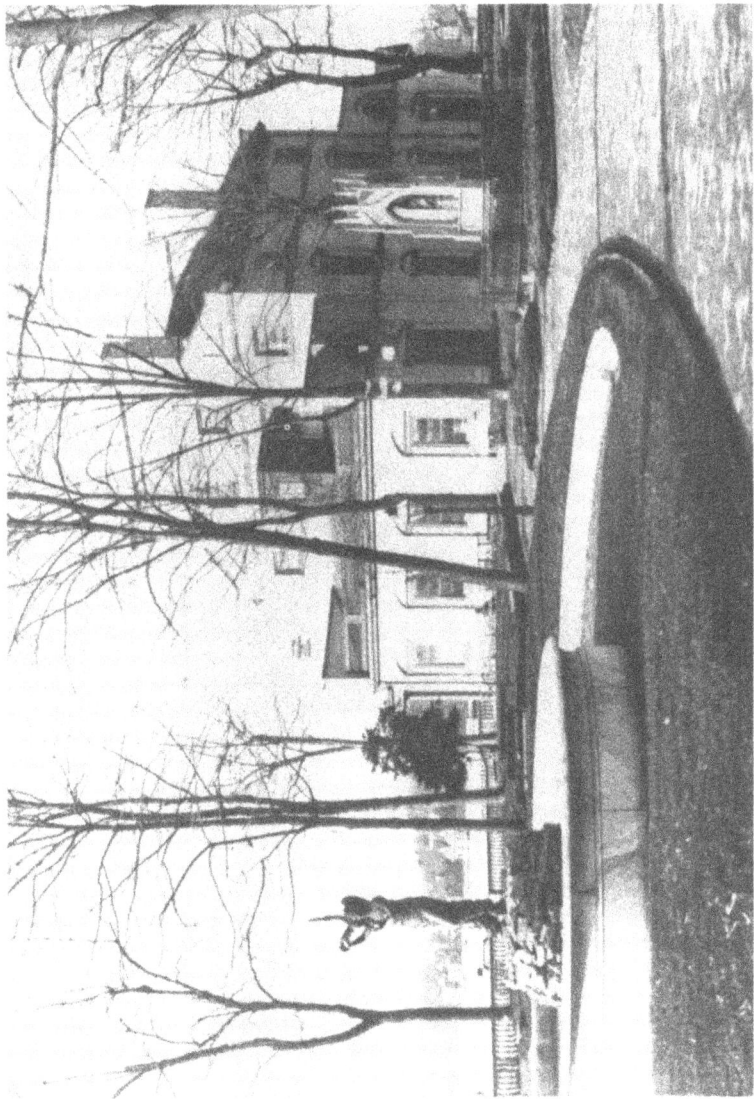

Engine House at Fairmount in the 1890s. View is to the northwest. Statue at left is a bronze copy of William Rush's wooden statue, ca. 1809, *Nymph and Bittern*. (The latter is a river bird on the girl's right shoulder.) Originally at the Centre Square water works, the wooden statue was moved to Fairmount in the 1820s and was there for many years before it deteriorated beyond repair. The bronze statue was cast in 1854. It is now in the Philadelphia Museum of Art. The gothic-spired monument near the Engine House is a memorial to Frederick Graff, the designer of the water works. It is still there. Courtesy of Germantown Historical Society.

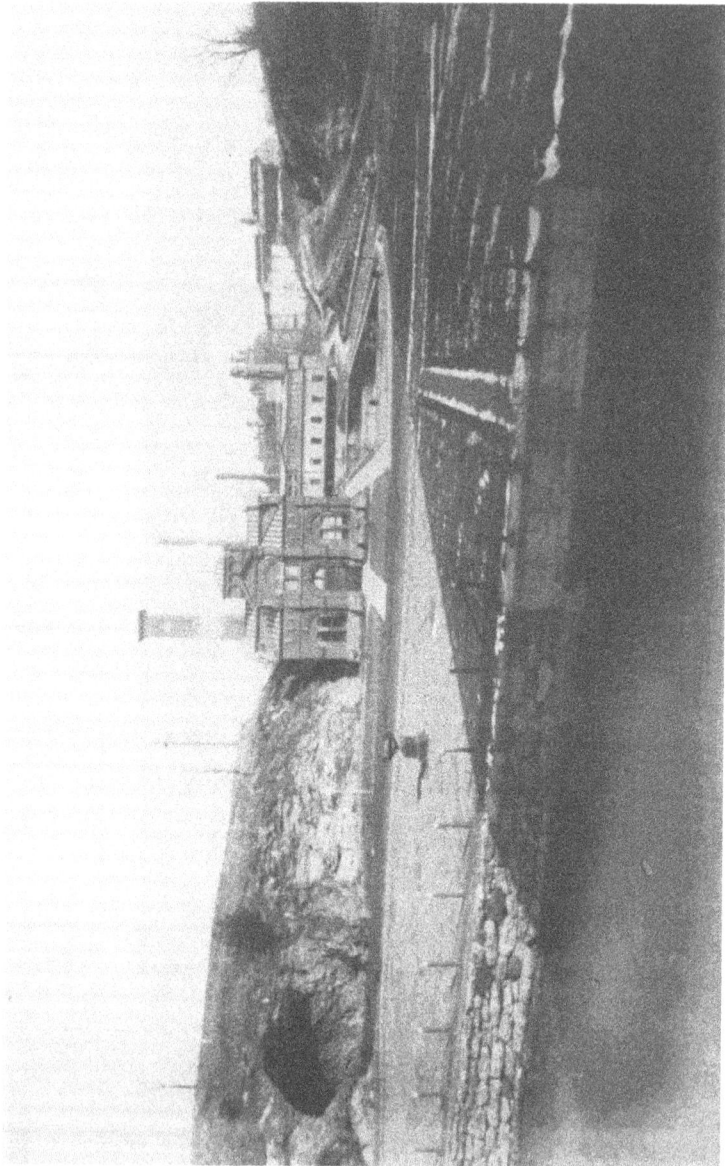

Spring Garden water works in the 1890s. Schuylkill river and water intake in foreground. Spring Garden built the works in 1844 when it was still a suburb of Philadelphia. The works were on the East River (Kelly) Drive just north of the Girard Avenue bridge. Courtesy of Germantown Historical Society.

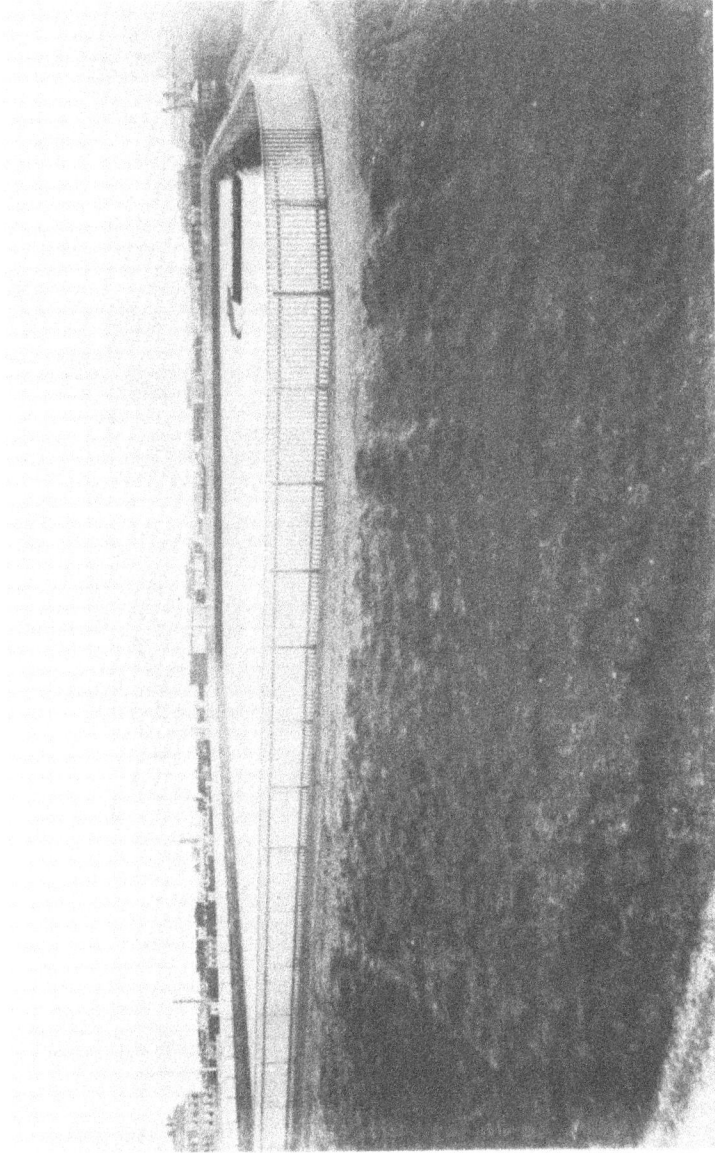

Spring Garden reservoir at 26th and Masters street in the 1890s. View is to the east. The reservoir had a capacity of approximately 13 million gallons. Courtesy of Germantown Historical Society.

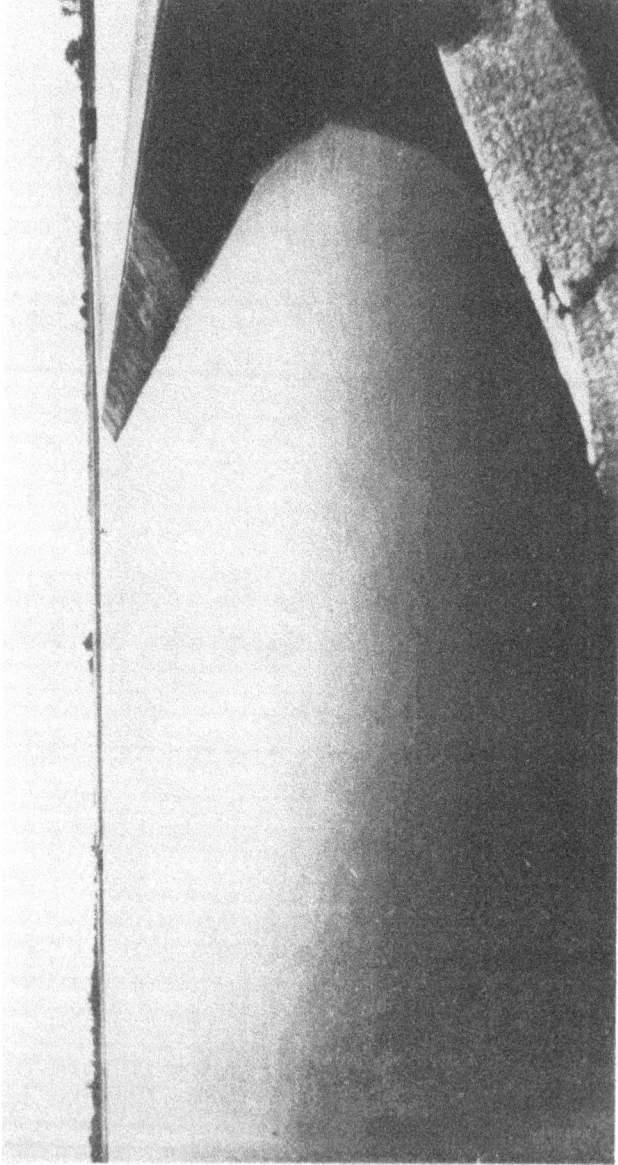

Second section of the East Park reservoir. Capacity was 396.4 million gallons. Total capacity of the reservoir's three sections was 688.6 million gallons. Reservoir was completed in 1889. This was part of the project to increase reserves and improve water quality by sedimentation. Courtesy of Germantown Historical Society.

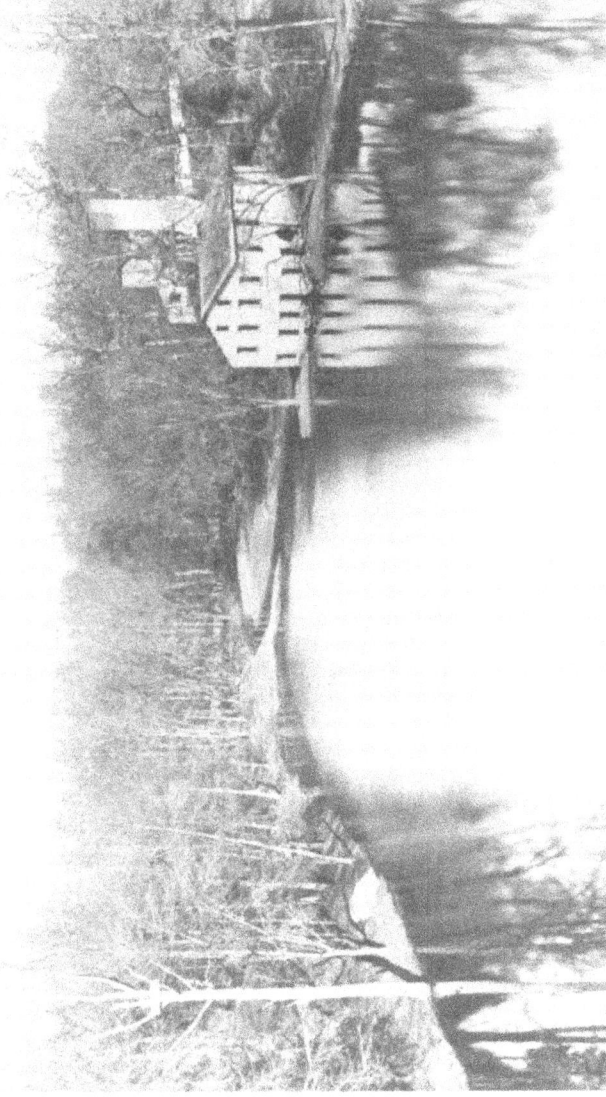

Pond and old water works at Germantown in the 1890s. The water source was a small stream that can be seen in the upper middle. The works closed down in 1872 when pollution from mills and factories upstream became too severe. Works were near Morris St. entrance to Lincoln Drive. Courtesy of Germantown Historical Society.

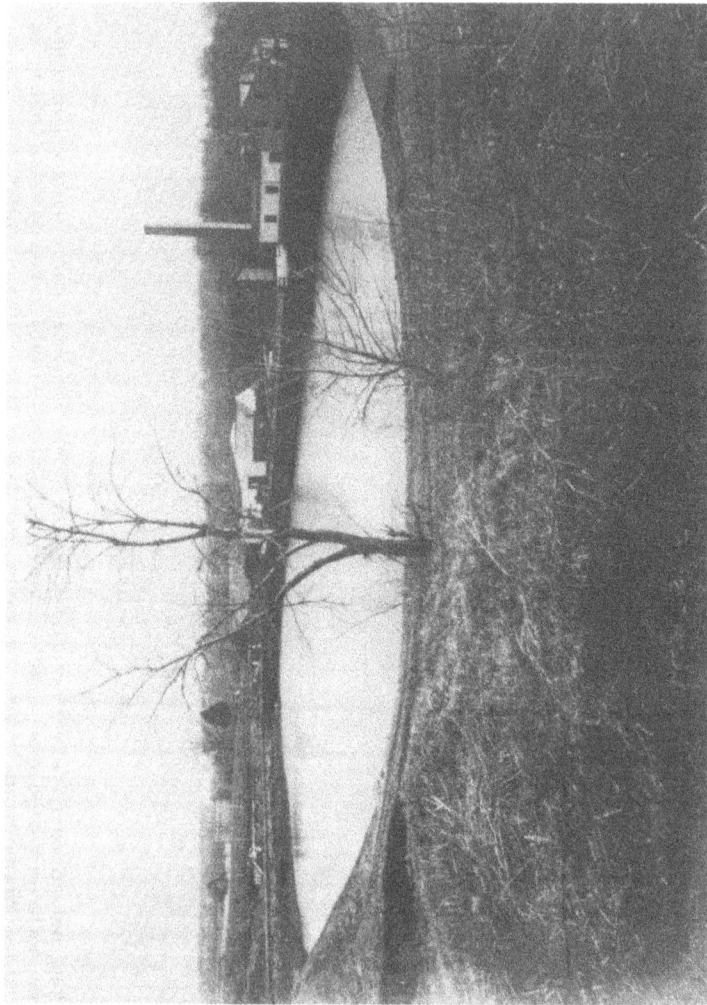

Reservoir at Chestnut Hill in 1890s near the present Gravers Lane station of SEPTA. View is to the east. Capacity was 5 million gallons. A standpipe with a capacity of 52,000 gallons was nearby. The main source of supply was a local spring. The works closed in 1910. Courtesy of Germantown Historical Society.

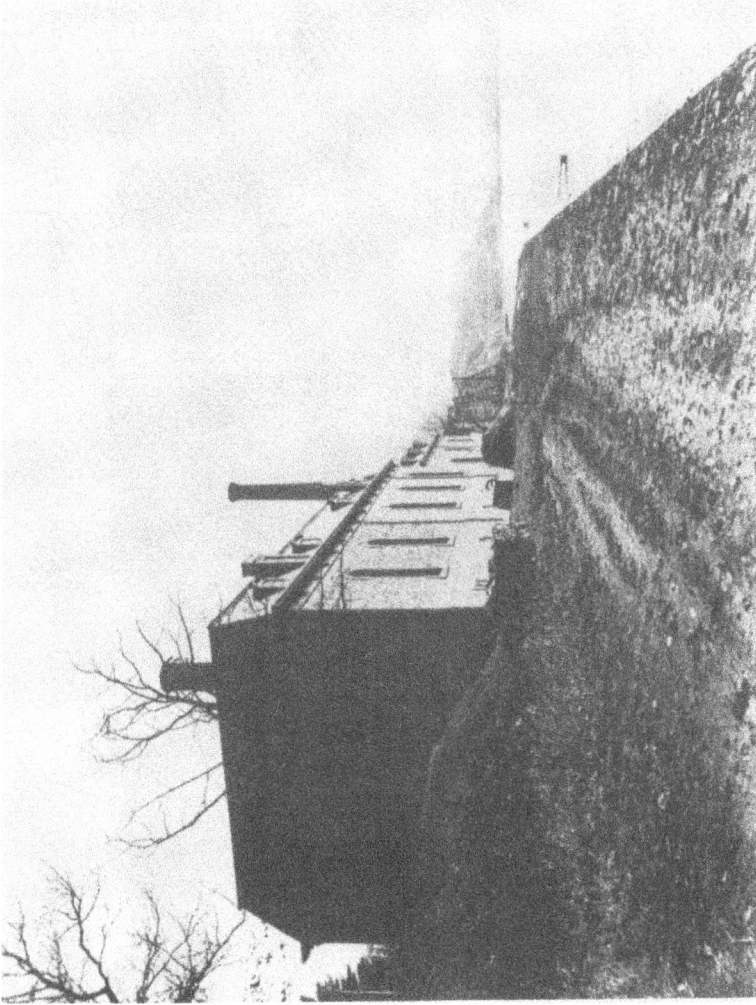

Pumping station at Roxborough in 1890s. View is to the south toward Manayunk. Courtesy of Germantown Historical Society.

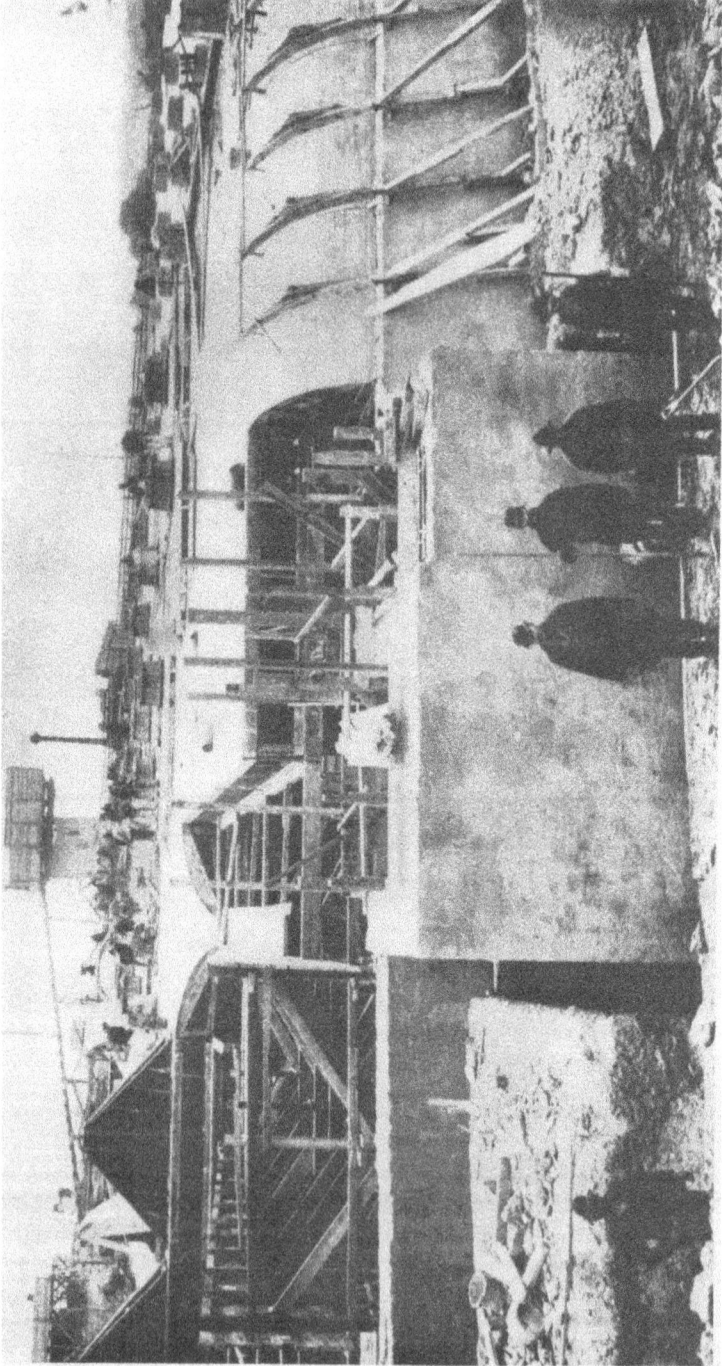

Filter beds under construction at Lower Roxborough in 1901. Courtesy of Historical Society of Pennsylvania.

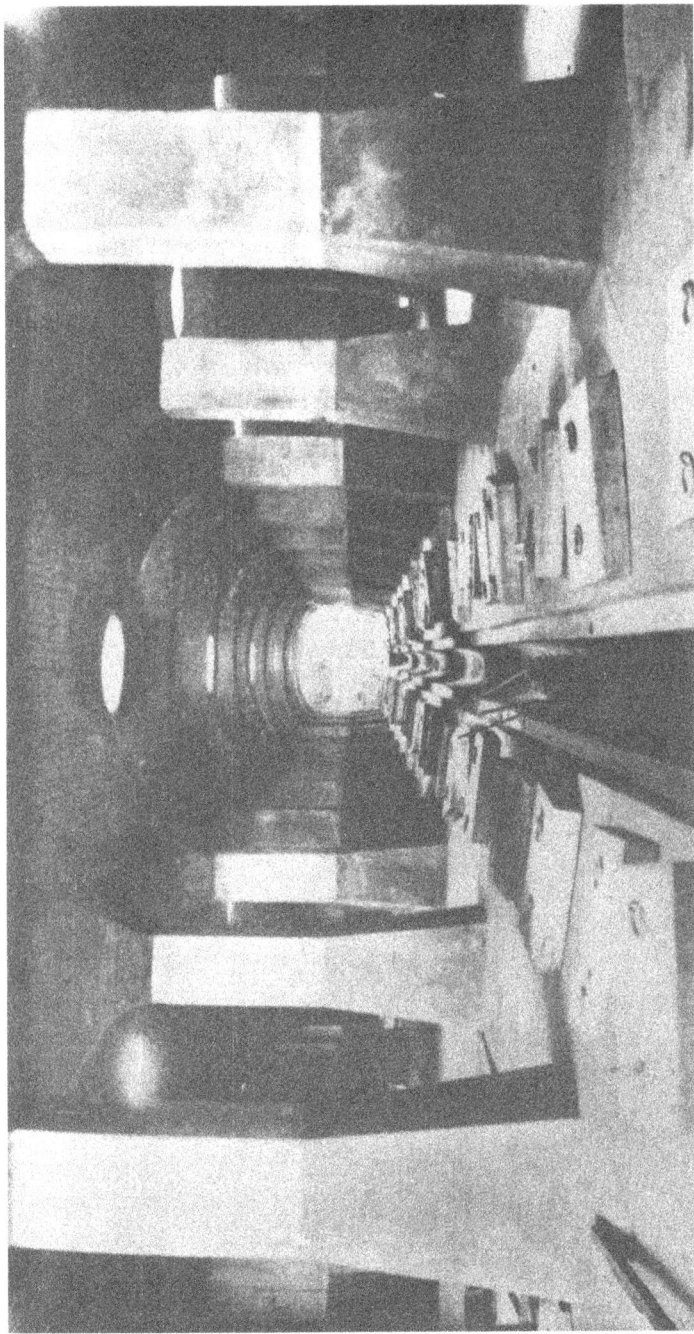

Interior of filter beds under construction at Lower Roxborough filters. Photo taken 1901. Courtesy of Historical Society of Pennsylvania.

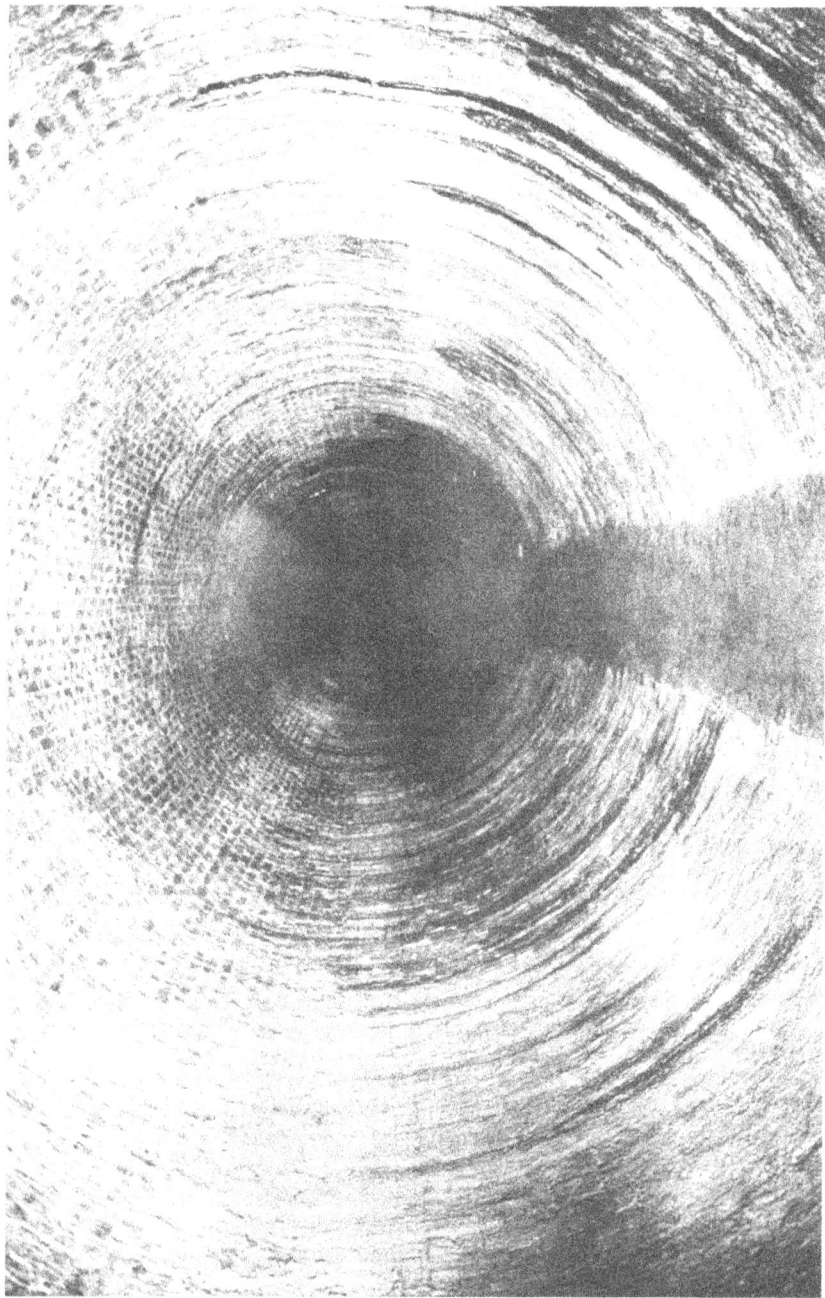

The controversial tunnel of Torresdale conduit during construction in 1904. Tunnel was 10 feet seven inches in diameter. One hundred feet underground and approximately 2½ miles long, the conduit ran from the Torresdale works to the relay pumping station at Lardner's Point in Frankfort. Some water from the outside seeped through the brickwork (stains on the walls and dark "path") when the conduit was empty; in use, leakage occurred in the other direction because the pressure was greater on the inside. This resulted in a small water loss, but it did not affect water safety for consumers. Courtesy of Historical Society of Pennsylvania.

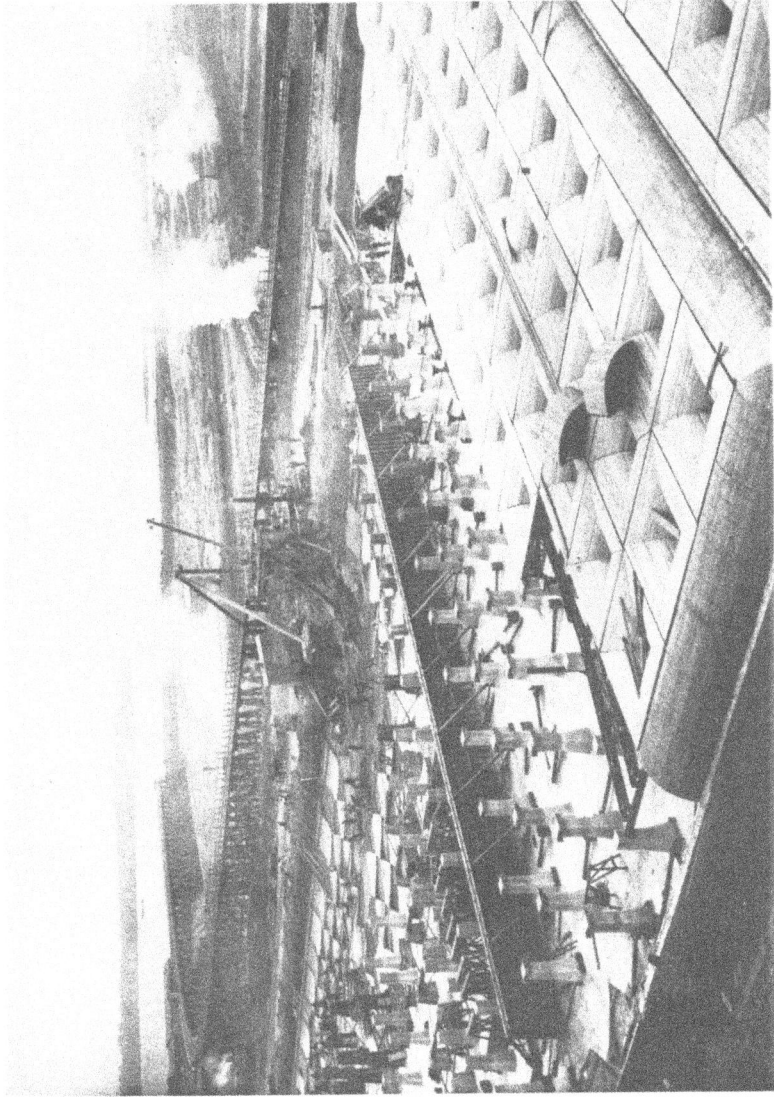

Filter beds under construction at Torresdale. Delaware River is in the background. Photo taken around 1904. Courtesy of Historical Society of Pennsylvania.

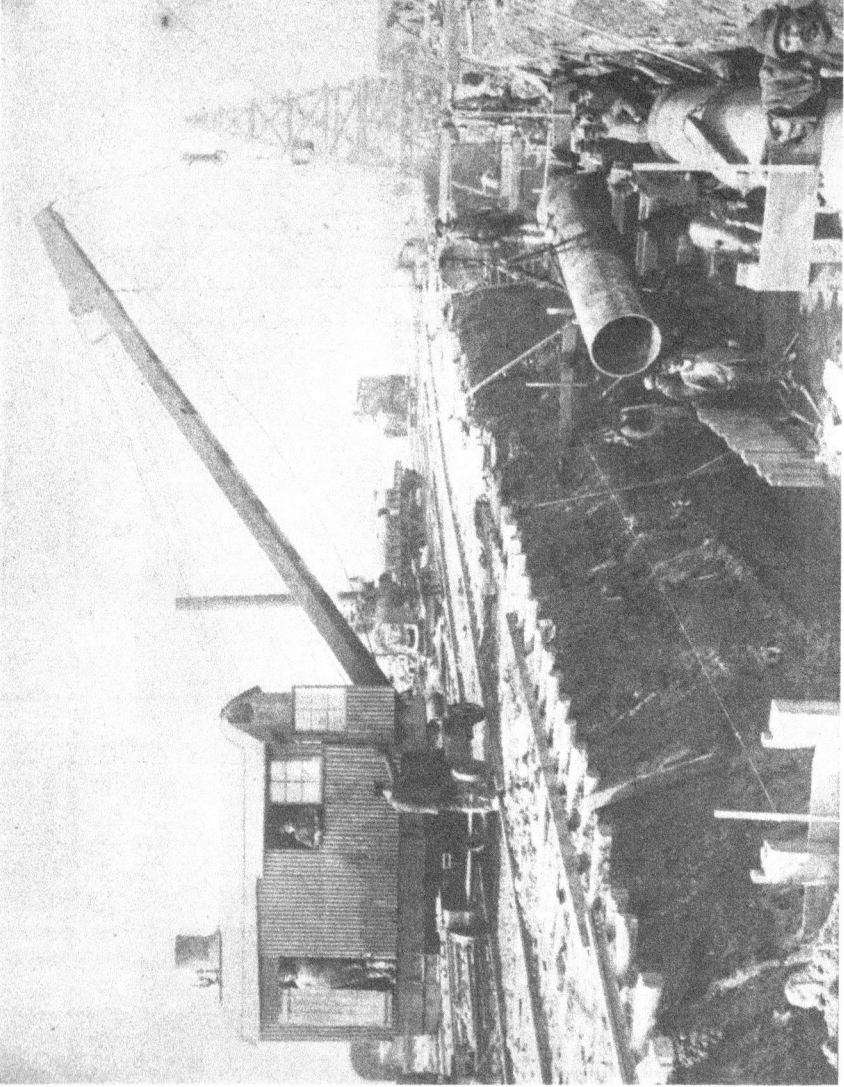

Laying pipe at Torresdale around 1904. Courtesy of Historical Society of Pennsylvania.

III. The Road toward Consensus

Getting money to pay for filtration was first on the agenda for water reformers in 1897. On 20 January delegates from the City Organizations' Filtration Committee and the Woman's Protective Health Association were in attendance when the joint finance committee of the councils met to consider the filtration plans. Unfortunately the councilmen voted 14-4 not to proceed further with the filtration plans until a court case was settled on the legality of the loan bill as well as another loan bill for $8 million that was passed earlier in 1896 for a new building for Central High School, a new Free Library building, and several other major projects. Some grumbling had been going on in the councils about all the spending, some of the criticism said to be politically motivated by Warwick's opponents who did not want to see him accomplish anything during his four years in office. But there were also valid questions about the debt limits, so the delay was not totally unexpected, but it was a disappointment nonetheless.[1]

In May a common court judge in Philadelphia ruled that the city could increase its indebtedness by the $11 million in the two loan bills. Opponents made an appeal to the state supreme court, but everyone in the mayor's office was confident that the common court ruling would be sustained. They were getting the loan items ready for council approval when the supreme court made its decision late in May. The city could increase its indebtedness, but it would have to prepare new legislation and the loans would have to be ap-

---

[1]*Public Ledger*, 21 January 1897.

proved by a referendum at a major election, the next one not
being until November.[2]

Thus more delays. With a second chance at a preparing a
laundry list of needed improvements, the councils added
more projects, raising the indebtedness in the bill to $12.2
million, a figure which was within the city's debt limit but
higher than the original one, as critics noted. The councils
also raised eyebrows when they dropped the plans for the
new library and shifted those $1.1 million dollars to a street
improvement item. They changed their minds on that
switch, but the episode reinforced the view that the new loan
bill was too unwieldy. Allow voters to make a decision on an
item-by-item basis, critics said. "If you compel the people to
take all or none, you will be surprised to see how many will
take nothing," one councilman warned. But the majority
decided to stick with the "all or none" approach.[3] This upset
the *Public Ledger*, which urged its readers to vote "no," even
though the paper supported most of the improvements in
the loan bill, including filtration.

The prospects were not bad, however, because the loan
had considerable backing. Dr. William Pepper, the provost of
the University of Pennsylvania, was interested in the library
project as well as filtration. Pepper was one of many prominent citizens who served on a promotion committee appointed by the mayor, and they talked at rallies aimed at a
variety of Philadelphians, from suburban matrons to Kensington workers on their lunch break.[4] The Democrats decided to oppose it as a party, but ironically this helped
because the Republicans countered by making it a party issue to see the bill passed, and the GOP enjoyed a top-heavy
majority of voters who could be turned out in large numbers
by formidable ward organizations.

On 3 November the bill carried by a margin of some
17,000, which showed that there was some voter dissatisfac-
tion since margins of 60,000 were the norm for bills the
GOP pushed, but the margin was healthy nonetheless. And

---

[2]Ibid., 1 June 1897.
[3]*Public Ledger*, 25 September 1897.
[4]For speeches by Pepper and others on the eve of voting, see *Public Ledger*, 1
November 1897.

so the loan was approved. Or at least the right to appropriate the money was approved. The rest was now up to the councils, who would have to prepare and pass bills for each of the projects.

The controversy over the large numbers of dollars in the loan bill did not do the cause of filtration much good because it raised again the nagging issue of exactly what filtration was going to cost the taxpayers. The councils had earmarked $3 million in the loan bill for filtration, a figure which was lower than the $3.5 million Trautwine estimated the cost would be based on actual consumption in 1896, but Trautwine was still hoping to get meters approved so the money would be enough if he was successful.

The $3 million figure was also close to the $3.4 million estimate that Allen Hazen had given in a report he had prepared for the Woman's Health Protective Association in 1896.[5] Hazen was a highly regarded engineer who had worked with the Lawrence experimental station and designed the slow sand filtration plant at Albany, New York, which was then the biggest of its kind in the country. The problem with Hazen's estimate was that it was not very realistic in the sense that he was projecting costs on ideal consumption, not actual consumption.

Hazen based his costs on a plant filtering 195 million gallons daily, which he admitted was "much less than now being used" (then 235 million gallons daily), but he felt that his figure was "ample for all purposes." Philadelphia, he said, was "using water in a most wasteful and extravagant manner and immediate measures should be taken to check such waste, and to reduce the consumption to a reasonable amount."[6] The introduction of meters could cut consumption and costs, he said. All of this was true, but taking into account the city's opposition to meters, Hazen's figures seemed folly.

In the fall of 1897 Trautwine released a report that was a good deal more realistic. No longer optimistic about saving

---

[5]Hazen, *A Practical Plan for Sand Filtration as a Means of Seeing a Better Water Supply for the City of Philadelphia* (1896), Historical Society of Pennsylvania library. Trautwine discusses Hazen's report in his own *Annual Report* (1896), 121-122 and includes a reprint of the report in Appendix N, 381-385.
[6]Hazen, *A Practical Plan*, 384.

money and water with meters, he said the city should expect
to spend between $8 and $10 million for a system capable of
filtering 400 million gallons daily, or the amount it appeared
the city would be consuming by the early 1900s.[7]

***

Given the sharply rising estimates, it is not surprising that
some members of the councils began to show renewed interest in the aqueduct idea. Instead of spending all those mil-
lions on improvements, they said, why not let a private
company supply us with pure water, especially since many of
them were then offering to do so. The most intriguing proposal was the one that Joseph Wharton had first suggested in
1891 without making any formal proposal to the city—and
then left more or less as a standing offer, Trautwine having
gone out to inspect his holdings in 1896.

Wharton was a wealthy Philadelphia financier and phi-
lanthropist who had made a fortune in mining and iron making and endowed the business school at the University of
Pennsylvania that bears his name. Around 1870 Wharton
became interested in growing sugar beets as another investment project, and he began buying up land in the area of
south central New Jersey known as the Pine Barrens.[8] The
beet project proved a bust because the top soil was too por-
ous, but the 120 square miles he owned by the 1890s turned
out to be valuable in other ways.

Or at least it offered potential value for its underground
water, the Pine Barrens being what John McPhee has called
"one of the greatest natural recharging areas in the world,"
with water beneath the sandy topsoil the equivalent of a lake
seventy five feet deep and a thousand miles in surface area.[9]
Wharton proposed to pump water from streams in his tract
to a reservoir he would build near Moorestown, some nine

[7]*Public Ledger*, 8 October 1897.
[8]Joanna Wharton Lippincott, *Biographical Memoranda concerning Joseph Wharton,
1826-1909* (Philadelphia, 1909), 52-53.
[9]McPhee, *The Pine Barrens* (New York, 1968), 14.

miles from Philadelphia. From there the water would go by pipe under the Delaware River to the city's reservoirs for distribution. A civil engineer who surveyed Wharton's property in 1891 estimated that his streams had a daily flow of some 385 million gallons, which was far in excess of what Philadelphia was then using. The water was exceptionally clean too, the engineer said, naturally filtered as it was by all the sand.[10]

Wharton admitted in 1891 that "the really difficult point in the plan will be to find terms sufficiently liberal to induce large and small capitalists to invest their money in an enterprise which, like all human undertakings, has its elements of risk, and at the same time moderate enough to be satisfactory to the city."[11] Apparently the point proved difficult indeed because Wharton never came up with a detailed proposal, so the city never really had an offer to consider.

However pure the Pine Barrens water may have been, its color was not all that attractive, which may have had something to do with the reason why Wharton's proposal never got backing. Except after rainfall when it was quite clear, the water in the Pine Barrens had a brown color like tea, from the iron deposits and the tannic acids of trees. McPhee says in summertime the water is usually "so dark that the riverbeds are obscured and while drifting along one has the feeling of being afloat a river of fast-moving ink."[12] A letter writer to the *Bulletin* in commenting favorably on Wharton's proposal admitted that the water had a "tawny color" and the "user needs to become accustomed to its looks."[13]

The biggest problem no doubt was that Wharton's holdings were in New Jersey, which meant that another state would be controlling Philadelphia's water supply—a point the head of the water bureau had noted with uneasiness in his annual report for 1891. To be sure, nothing prohibited the transfer, but the New Jersey legislature in 1905 passed a law banning the sale of water to another state unless it received official approval. Even if New Jersey had approved,

---

[10]The engineer's report is included in Board of Health, *Annual Report* (1891), Appendix H.
[11]Letter was dated 17 June 1891 and reprinted in Lippincott, *Joseph Wharton*, 54-56.
[12]McPhee, *Pine Barrens*, 16-17.
[13]Letter reprinted in Lippincott, *Joseph Wharton*, 53-54.

Philadelphians themselves may have had second thoughts, given the risks inherent in such an arrangement.[14]

At any rate, a consortium calling itself the Schuylkill Valley Water Company had a deal that seemed more workable. They would supply Philadelphia with 400 million gallons of water daily from upper Schuylkill by building a series of dams from Reading to Norristown that would hold some 18 billion gallons. The company would also build filtering plants and pipe the water to the city's pumping stations. In addition the company would build a filtering plant on the Delaware, which would supply the northeast section of the city. The job would be completed within three years of the signing of the contract, the company said. It was also willing to pay penalties if it failed to meet its time schedule. In fifty years the company would turn the system over to the city. In return the city would pay the company $1.5 million a year, or approximately the same amount the city was taking in from water bill receipts.

An irresistible scheme for the city, company spokesmen said, but few others seemed to feel that way, least of all Trautwine. The company could not build those dams, he said, without all kinds of litigation problems since they would require extensive flooding of the countryside. Even if they could, the dams would be too shallow to hold the amount of water needed on a daily basis when consumption reached 400 million gallons.

What bothered Trautwine most were the financial aspects of the plan. To be sure, the city would eventually own the system, but Trautwine felt fifty annual payments of $1.5 million or a total of $75 million was a bit steep for a plant that would cost the company $10 million to build. It also meant that the city would tie up all its revenue from water bill receipts. Even having to pay interest on a bond issue, it would be much cheaper for the city to raise the monies nec-

---

[14]The law in 1905 apparently came in response to efforts of a private company to sell water from the Passaic River to New York, and the courts upheld the state in the appeal that followed. Ironically, it was not until 1981 that New Jersey passed legislation to protect the watershed in the Pine Barrens. The bill covers approximately 1 million acres in the Pinelands National Reserve, a recreation area that was created by a federal law in 1978. It includes much of Wharton's former holdings.

essary for construction through a bond issue. No, Trautwine concluded, the proposal made no sense at all for the city.[15]

The mayor said the same thing—as did the chairmen of the joint committee of the councils' finance committee, the County Medical Society, and the City Organizations' Filtration Committee. The Civic Club, a women's club, also noted its disapproval, and it held a special meeting on 21 February to organize opposition.[16]

But the Schuylkill Valley Water Company bill stayed very much alive, thanks to the efforts of a handful of councilmen led by Edward W. Patton, a select councilman from the 27th ward in Southwest Philadelphia and an influential Republican regular who had a flourishing electrical contracting business. Patton and his friends were Penrose supporters who were becoming more obstructionist in their attitude toward the Warwick administration. If the mayor did not like the Schuylkill Valley Water Company bill, that was just the bill to pass, or so their attitude seemed to indicate. In the councils, however, they talked only about the positive side of the Schuylkill Valley Water Bill, particularly that the city would not have to float loans for construction costs. Given the controversy over the loan monies, this was not a small point in the minds of many councilmen.

First Patton and his colleagues had to block the passage of a bill for the filtration plan from the loan money, and they succeeded in doing that early in 1898.[17] Then they went to work on the Schuylkill Valley Water Company bill. Once a head count indicated that they had the necessary votes needed in the select council, they pushed the bill through by a vote of 22-14 on 1 March. The bill then went to the common council where the friends of Patton in that chamber also seemed to have enough votes for passage.

When the common council met on 10 March, opponents of the bill offered a motion to postpone indefinitely any action on it. When that failed, councilman Walter Stevenson,

[15]*Public Ledger*, 24 February 1898; full report in Bureau of Water, *Annual Report* (1897), 72ff.
[16]*Public Ledger*, 1, 14, 26 February 1898; *North American*, 2 March 1898; *Inquirer*, 22 February 1898.
[17]Ibid., 28 January 1898; 25 February 1898.

an independent Republican from the 32nd ward in North Philadelphia, requested permission from the chair to speak, a move that startled everyone since Stevenson had been in the council for over a year and never asked to speak before. Stevenson seemed clearly nervous as he began to talk, and some of the oldtimers made sarcastic remarks, which made him even more uncomfortable. But his voice quickly became louder and more confident, and it was clear this was going to be no ordinary speech.

Stevenson pounded his desk to silence his hecklers. "This is the first time I have ever spoken," he said, as the chamber grew quieter,

and I sincerely hope that the words I speak will have some effect. The statement I make here today, I make in the name of decency and honesty. In the name of the citizens of Philadelphia and of my ward I want it distinctly understood I was elected as an honest man. This is what I am here for. I have had two or three chances to be made a damn fool of. I deplore the fact, Mr. President, that the statement is made that Councils are rotten,

he said, making reference to all the remarks in the press against the water bill.

Mr. President, to come right down to the point I desire to take up, I want to say, Mr. President, as an honest man and a man of veracity, I have been offered $5,000 to vote for this bill, and I want an investigation, Mr. President. I want to say that the remark was made to me that every man that was voting for this bill was getting $1,000 to $5,000, and I would get the greatest amount offered for a vote. I say this rottenness ought to cease right now, and I call on the councils of the city of Philadelphia to stop it today. I am willing to go before any tribunal and prove what I have said.

After a moment of stunned silence, one of Patton's lieutenants, councilman William Von Osten, shouted, "The gentleman says he was offered $5,000 to vote for this bill. I would ask the member how much did he want?" An opponent of the water bill shouted back at Von Osten, "How much did you get for the support of the bill?" As more shouting matches started, councilman Seeds quickly came to the front of the chamber and requested the indefinite postponement of any action on the bill. Patton and his friends tried mightily to defeat the motion, but it passed, 67-62.[18]

Stevenson was a member of a family that owned a home construction company in North Philadelphia. It seems he had been offered money several times at the company office at 30th and Diamond streets by Peter E. Smith, a well-known local politico and member of the Republican city committee for the neighboring 29th Ward. Smith was so casual about his bribe offers that he even discussed them in front of one of Stevenson's brothers, James, who was also a member of the firm. "What do you think of Walter?" Smith was quoted as saying. "He has a chance to make $5,000, and he is going to throw it over his shoulder."[19]

Smith denied everything, but district attorney George S. Graham went ahead with preparing charges. Graham was a tough-minded and highly regarded independent Republican who was in his sixth term of office. Graham and Warwick were old friends, and Graham had been something of a mentor for the mayor, Warwick having served under Graham in the district attorney's office earlier in his career. Like Warwick, Graham had no love for the Schuylkill water bill and even less for the machine politicians who pushed it.

At the formal arraignment of Smith, Graham subpoenaed the entire joint committee on water, a move which raised some eyebrows, but it was soon clear what he was up to when he got select councilman Louis J. Walker of the 12th ward on the stand to give testimony. Walker was one of Philadelphia's lesser lights in the councils, a mousey, slow-witted fellow who did more or less what he was told to do and little else. Clearly nervous after he was sworn in, Walker stoutly denied that he had taken any money. Despite Walker's refusal to admit anything, Graham remained pleasant as he questioned Walker from his seat. He thumbed through some papers on his desk and let the witness ramble on. As the *Inquirer* described the episode, suddenly[20]

Graham the persuasive changed into Graham the terrible. "Now

[18]*Inquirer*, 11 March 1898.
[19]Ibid., 16 March 1898.
[20]Ibid., 24 March 1898.

sir," he thundered, jumping up with a bound, and glaring eyes flashing power and determination, and finger pointed threateningly. "Now sir, I want the truth. You may as well tell the truth now, and I mean you shall." The witness trembled perceptibly. The judge found on the same line: "With God as your judge, answer me the truth. You owe it to yourself." "Now Mr. Walker," again broke in Mr. Graham. "I will give you one minute to reflect. Then I will ask you once more, and I want you to tell the truth."

The district attorney's tactics completely broke down Walker, who after the minute of silence admitted that he had been lying. Yes, he was offered a bribe to approve the Schuylkill bill in the water committee. Two in fact: one for $5,000 from councilman Byram and one for $500 from councilman Seger. Yes, he had taken the $500 actually offered him. "How long after the committee's report was in was the money paid to you?" asked Graham.

"I think it was the next day."
"The next day after the committee's report was in?"
"Yes, sir."
"Who paid the money? Tell it straight out. Who paid the money?"
"Mr. Seger."
"Where did he pay you the money?"
"In his building."
"Where is his building?"
"Opposite here."
(Judge Bregy) "What is his building?"
"Tavern."
(Judge Bregy) "You were in there and it was paid to you by him?"
"Yes, sir."
(Mr. Graham) "Did he tell you where he got the money?"
"No, sir."
"How was it paid to you—in money or in a check?"
"Money."

Yes, he knew of at least one other councilman who accepted a bribe: councilman Edwin Smith of the 11th ward, who was paid $500 by Seger at the same time. Yes, he imagined others were bribed, but he did not know their names. And so the testimony went on.[21]

---

[21]Ibid.

The name of Nelson Green, the chief lobbyist for the Schuylkill Valley Water Company, was mentioned frequently during the investigation, but Green was smart enough to stay well backstage when any money was handed over to councilmen. Graham felt he had enough on Green anyway to indict him, but the case was later dropped for lack of evidence. With denials to Walker's story by the councilmen he named and no other witnesses, Graham did not bother to charge Walker, and the case against Peter Smith fell through on a technicality. So in the end there were no convictions. Graham was angry and disappointed, but the outcome was not surprising given the difficulties of prosecuting these cases.

In any event, it is surprising that no one had blown the whistle on the bribers before Stevenson. In his testimony during the investigation, for example, Robert R. Bringhurst, a member of the common council from Center City and co-chairman of the joint water committee, admitted that Green had talked about bribes when he came to see the councilman shortly after the bill was introduced. Referring to Bringhurst's colleagues in the councils, Green said "I know some of them will have to be seen and fixed. I wish you to find out who these gentlemen are and what they want, and I will look for the balance." Bringhurst warned Green not to make him any proposition because, he said, "On questions of public interest I am very apt to leak like a sieve."[22] Green did not approach him again, which may explain why Bringhurst did not speak up when the bill was moving along. No doubt the lobbyists kept away from Bringhurst's friends too, and those who had taken money were not talking. No one apparently would have talked had not Smith made the mistake of approaching Stevenson.

It is impossible to piece together all the behind-the-scenes events related to this episode, but from the sequence of events on the day of Stevenson's speech it appears that Seeds knew what Stevenson was going to say since he moved so quickly once Stevenson had finished. Moreover, Seeds said he had additional evidence to substantiate Stevenson's

---

[22]Ibid.

charges, news that seemed to provide an extra jolt to a stunned council.

The sources of the evidence turned out to be Dr. William Pepper, Frank Firth, the president of the City Organizations' Filtration Committee, and Anne Scribner, the president of the Woman's Health Protective Association. When they appeared at a council hearing, Pepper said he believed improper methods were used to push the bill but admitted he had no knowledge of bribery or any attempts at bribery.[23] Angry as he had been at Nelson Green, Firth had no proof either.[24]

All that Scribner could offer in the way of incriminating evidence was that Green had promised her a generous donation for her association's playground in Kensington if she would use her influence to see that his company's ordinance was passed.[25] Seeds may well have known on the day of Stevenson's revelation that Pepper and the others had no hard evidence about bribes, but his bluff—if it was that—proved effective because it helped to get the postponement motion passed and that in effect killed the bill.

In any case, it is highly unlikely that the Schuylkill Valley Water Company scheme would have been implemented even if it had passed the common council. Mayor Warwick had said he would veto the bill, and its backers did not appear to have enough votes to override that veto. The lobbyists might have tried to buy some more votes, of course, but that would not necessarily have guaranteed passage, given the controversy. No doubt district attorney Graham also would have been out scouring his contacts for some evidence of bribery to stop the bill that way if all else failed.

As for the bill itself, there was nothing inherently wrong with the idea of a private company assuming a lease for public services. Bringhurst, Seeds, and many of their friends

[23]Ibid., 23 March 1898. Pepper was gravely ill at the time but obviously still active in water reform, and he worked to keep the newspapers in line against the bill; Francis Newton Thorpe, *William Pepper* (New York, 1904), 502-503. For more on Pepper and his papers at the University of Pennsylvania, see Note on Sources.
[24]Early in February Nelson Green had sent Firth a copy of his water company's proposal. Firth replied that he was familiar with it, but did not understand why Green would expect the city to turn over the water works to a private company. "Everything you proposed to do, the city can itself do more cheaply and better than you can." Firth to Green, 3 February 1898, letterbook, Firth papers.
[25]*Inquirer*, 23 March 1898.

in fact supported the leasing of the city gas works to a private company in the fall of 1897, a controversial deal at the time, but it apparently was working out well for the city when the Schuylkill Valley Water Company bill came up—a fact that was not lost on its supporters who made references to the earlier gas ordinance in their speeches. If private enterprise can serve us gas, why can't it serve us water, they asked. Before the scandal broke, the argument seemed reasonable enough, but the gas works and the water works were really not the same in important respects. The water works, for example, required relatively few employees so the personnel costs were not as high as they were with the gas works. The water works were also actually making money—over $1 million a year after expenses—and this made leasing less attractive.

In any case, the city could ill afford to waste time in its fight against typhoid. Conditions were getting no better—in fact they seemed to be getting a good deal worse. On 16 November 1897, around the time the push began for the Schuylkill Valley Water Company bill, a crew flushing the interceptor sewer put too much water into it and the sewer backed up and overflowed into the Schuylkill directly above the Queen Lane pumping station. Apparently the workers did not report the accident promptly, and the pumps were stopped at Queen Lane only after polluted water was seen in the reservoir at 4 p.m., or about two hours after the overflow began.

At 9 p.m. when the water department received word of bad-tasting water from the district supplied by the Fairmount works, it stopped pumping at all the stations south of Queen Lane, and it did not resume pumping until the afternoon of the next day. The bacteria count in the reservoir water was high, but this did not necessarily mean it was dangerously contaminated because it had been raining for several days, and a high bacteria count was normal during rainy conditions when extra amounts of dirt and leaves were in the water. The incubation period for typhoid was several weeks. All that the board of health could do was wait and hope for the best.[26]

---

[26] A complete report on the episode was prepared by Dr. Alexander C. Abbott, chief

By the third week of December it was clear that the reservoirs had indeed been contaminated. The number of cases had doubled, to 400 for the month compared to 200 for November. All but three of the city's thirty-eight wards showed an increase, the worst hit being the seven wards served by the Queen Lane pumping station where 53 percent of the cases were reported. In January the board of health expected the number of cases to decline since anyone infected by the 16th November overflow should have become ill by then. But in fact things got worse. The number of reported cases jumped to 860 that month or twice the total number reported in December. In February the number of new cases dropped a bit to 670 and then fell sharply to 362 in March before it fell back to a more or less average normal figure of 196 in April.

Although no one knew for sure why the epidemic lasted so long, the great increase in cases in districts served by the Roxborough pumping station at the city's northern limits seemed to support what Ludlow and Hartshorne said in the 1880s—that Montgomery County was contributing to the city's health problem. In the spring of 1898 the board of health sent some of its staff out to take a look. In Lower Merion Township a number of small streams meandered through Bryn Mawr and Rosemont and other nearby communities before forming a larger stream called Mill Creek that flowed down the steep ravines in Penn Valley to the Schuylkill.

The inspectors were especially interested in Mill Creek because the Roxborough pumping station was just a short distance below on the opposite side of the river. They found a number of small textile mills and factories like Seth Humphrey's Fairview Mill where a privy was located directly over the creek. At the Thomas Clegg carpet mill an abandoned mill race which flowed into Mill Creek served as an open cesspool for a half a dozen water closets used by employees; and another half dozen houses for workers and their families also had their privies near the mill race and the discharges washed down the bank and into the water. The

of the bacteriological division of the board of health. It was included in the *Annual Report* (1897), 176-184.

owners of the mill thought the sand that silted up the mouth of the mill race as it flowed into the creek purified the water, but the inspectors considered the efficiency of the sand as a filter to be "doubtful" at best.[27]

As a further insult to Philadelphia sensibilities, that summer a dead horse was discovered in the river above the Roxborough pumping station. Apparently it had floated into the Schuylkill from Plymouth Creek. Blaming the horse, Mount Airy residents complained about the taste of their water and went to the chief of the Mount Airy reservoir, but he said the water they were getting at the time came from the Roxborough reservoir. In any case, the horse was not within the city limits, and the state board of health had to be contacted to remove it. By the time that office had been reached, the bloated carcass had floated down past the pumping station to the Flat Rock dam, where city workers quickly pulled it out of the water.[28]

What was disconcerting about all this casual pollution was the awareness that a single individual had been responsible for the epidemic in Plymouth, Pennsylvania, in 1885 in which over a thousand of the town's 8,000 residents became ill and 114 died.[29] In that episode a man ill with typhoid had dumped his bedpan excreta in the snow outside his cabin all winter. Typhoid bacilli can survive even freezing temperatures and when the weather thawed, melting snows washed the virulent microbes into a nearby stream and infected Plymouth's water supply. No one believed that the dead horse or any of the privies along Mill Creek had been responsible for the most recent outbreak of typhoid in Philadelphia, but the threat was always there, given the lack of filtration.

It is difficult to say how many Philadelphians drank tap

[27]Bureau of Water, *Annual Report* (1898), 160.
[28]*Inquirer*, 7 July 1898. It was surprising that only Mount Airy residents complained since residents of Roxborough, Manayunk, and Germantown were also getting the same water. (The Roxborough pumps did not stop while the horse was in the river.) The Germantowners and others may have been inured to the taste.
[29]Stuart Galishoff, "Triumph and Failure: The American Response to the Urban Water Supply Problem, 1860-1923," in Martin V. Melosi, ed., *Pollution and Reform in American Cities, 1870-1930* (Austin, Texas, 1983), 43-44.
   The Plymouth Creek just mentioned is in suburban Montgomery County. The town Plymouth is on the Susquehanna River near Wilkes-Barre.

water at home. To be sure, tap water was also used for cook-ing and washing, but the *Public Ledger* was forever reminding its readers to boil their tap water whenever there was a se-rious outbreak of typhoid, something the paper would not have bothered to do, it would seem, if its readers never drank any. The city's most ardent boosters for filtration were the middle-class suburbanites in Germantown which sug-gests that they drank the water too—and apparently they did not like having to boil water to drink it. Protective mea-sures like this "ought not to be needed," Hartshorne said in his 1889 pamphlet, and he felt it was irresponsible for the city to make such measures necessary since many people, "especially among the poor, cannot or will not use" them.[30]

Well water was also available—at least in some neigh-borhoods. By the 1890s nearly all the wells had been filled in downtown between Vine and South Streets because of ground pollution, and the board of health was constantly ordering others that it considered a health hazard to be filled in. In some suburban districts, though, wells apparently could be quite safe. Cornelius Weygandt, an essayist and popular English professor at the University of Pennsylvania, writing in the 1930s remembered moving into a house on Wissahickon Avenue in Germantown in 1900 which had a deep well that his family used into the 1920s "when the city water failed us." The Weygandts stopped using it then only because they "could no longer find a plumber's man willing to go down to clean out a section of pump that had rotted and fallen into the bottom."[31]

Wells were especially popular in Germantown in the late nineteenth century because the city water was so bad, but there were risks involved with wells there—and in nearby Chestnut Hill and Wyndmoor where you would expect to have very safe ground water, given the low population den-sity. As proof of the potential threat, the board of health found nine wells in those communities to be unsafe and one "suspicious" when it did routine testing in 1898. In the ma-jority of samples, the board noted that the water was "clear,

[30]Hartshorne, *Our Water Supply*, 18.
[31]Weygandt, *Philadelphia Folks: Ways and Institutions in and about the Quaker City* (New York, 1938), 224.

colorless and odorless, and consequently gave no sensible evidence of pollution," news that must have been unsettling indeed to well owners and to anyone else who drank well water at the time.[32]

In Chestnut Hill some residents were also drinking local water, from a spring that fed the old Chestnut Hill works that were built back in the days when the community was an independent suburb. In 1854 Philadelphia annexed neighboring suburbs in Philadelphia County, and Chestnut Hill became part of the city.[33] The works were near the Gravers Lane station of the Reading line in Chestnut Hill. Water was pumped from the spring there into a small pond-like reservoir and then to an impressive stone standpipe (still there) that towered over the neighborhood. A water main ran to the tank from the Mount Airy reservoir and pumping station, but that apparently was opened only when water in the Chestnut Hill supply ran dangerously low and that may not have happened frequently—on only three days in 1876, for an example from earlier years. The water bureau seemed to consider this noteworthy enough to mention since the information was not a regular part of the annual report. The news in the 1890s that wells in Chestnut Hill could be polluted must have worried the water bureau since it obviously meant that spring water was vulnerable—and Chestnut Hill would not be the only community affected because water from the works was occasionally piped into Mount Airy reservoir. To be sure, the water pumped in Chestnut Hill was a relatively tiny amount (195,804 gallons pumped daily in 1884, for example, compared to 3,696,729 a day for the Roxborough pumping station), but even that amount could cause a major epidemic if the typhoid was in the water.

You could buy a glass of spring water from street vendors, as we see three men doing at 5th and Market streets in the 1890s in a photograph in *Still Philadelphia,* a photographic history of the city from 1890 to 1940.[34] "Pure Spring Water Direct from Delaware County," says the sign on the back of

---

[32]Board of Health, *Annual Report* (1898), 145-155.
[33]For the consolidation movement and the new city charter, see my article cited in Chapter I, n. 3.
[34]Frederic M. Miller, Morris J. Vogel, Allen F. Davis, *Still Philadelphia: A Photographic History, 1890-1940* (Philadelphia, 1983), 20.

the cart, and no doubt the vendor did a brisk business at his downtown corner.

The city business directories in the 1890s list a half dozen or so suppliers, and many more—like our nameless vendor in *Still Philadelphia*—were no doubt unlisted. Given all the problems of keeping a supply of bottled water and the added cost, it is doubtful that a significant number of Philadelphians drank it every day. And there was no guarantee either that the bottled water was safe since there were no codes for the product in those days.

And so it appeared that filtration was the only solution— and by the summer of 1898 even the councils were leaning that way. In July they asked Trautwine to update his earlier reports and submit some new recommendations, and by early October he had a lengthy report ready for review. In Trautwine's opinion the critical issue was still waste. According to his estimates, over 60 percent of the city's water was going down the drain unused, and filtering wasted water would cost the city over $7 million compared to around $2.3 for filtration plants that processed the water actually used.

To reduce the waste, Trautwine recommended meters for all manufacturing plants. He also wanted meters for homeowners who were found to be wasting water by willful neglect or faulty plumbing. Only around 20 percent of homeowners were considered to be in this category, Trautwine said, but he still felt that meters were a good way to help keep costs down for the other 80 percent of responsible water users who were paying indirectly for the wasted water. There might be some "hardships" he said for the "small minority" but it would only be a "temporary inconvenience of putting its plumbing in order and unlearning its habit of wastefulness."[35]

Trautwine recommended slow sand filters for all the pumping stations except for the district served by the Queen Lane works. There the city would have to make do with a mechanical filter because sand filters took up much more space and the land costs were high where the filters would

---

[35]Appendix 3, Journal of the Common Council (6 October 1898-30 March 1899), 45. The appendix also includes Trautwine's report and Thompson's reaction to it, as well as a covering letter from the mayor to the councils when the report was submitted.

have to be located—in a booming residential district in East Falls near Germantown. As to the relative merits of the different systems, Trautwine refused to make any comments, saying that he never had a chance to test them. In fact he believed that no system should be installed until an experimental station was built. Spend money on meters and an experimental station first, he told the councilmen. "Certainly with one such model plant in operation, the public would promptly insist on the extension of the meter system and of filtration to the rest of the city, and the water problem would be solved."[36] If nothing else, Trautwine was consistent.

The head of the department of public works, Thomas Thompson, was not particularly happy with the preoccupation with waste and meters that the report reflected. Thompson admitted that there was "great waste," but he also said that he was "unable to convince himself that there is a waste of 160 gallons per capita per day" as Trautwine had claimed in his report.[37] Per capita figures were not accurate indicators, he said, because manufacturers used great quantities of water, and cities like Philadelphia simply consumed more water than others with less industry.

Thompson was also not happy about Trautwine's recommendation for a mechanical filter at Queen Lane. Although he was willing to go along with it, Thompson was skeptical about the effectiveness of mechanical filters, and he worried too about possible problems with adding chemicals to the water, a worry that many contemporaries including some physicians shared with him.

What Thompson really wanted to do, as he told the councils at a meeting of the water committee shortly after they received the report, was to reduce greatly the dependence on the Schuylkill River—which then supplied over 90 percent of the city's water—by increasing the supply of water from the Delaware River which was much less polluted, at least upstream in Northeast Philadelphia. A new pumping station with slow sand filters could be built at Torresdale, which was within the city limits but still a rural area where

---

[36]Ibid.
[37]Ibid., 9; *Public Ledger*, 12 October 1898.

the flow of the Delaware was much cleaner. With more water coming from the Delaware, Thompson said the city would not need to build a mechanical filter at Queen Lane. His proposal was sound, but it was not the same as Trautwine's, and it underlined the differences even within the administration.

Differences notwithstanding, Trautwine's report at least helped to move things along in the sense that issues were aired and consensus reached in some areas. There was almost unanimous opinion in the councils and the press, for example, that meters were not the way to solve the water problem. In urging the councils to oppose meters, particularly for homes, the *Public Ledger* picked up on Thompson's criticism of Trautwine's figures by noting that[38]

It is not at all certain that there is an "enormous" waste as it is alleged by some. It does not follow because there is a larger per capita use of water here than in other cities, that the excess is due to waste. It is just as likely to be because the householder is more active in the work of cleanliness. Instead of lamenting because the per capita consumption in this city is greater than elsewhere, it seems rather a matter for congratulations, and far from seeking means to secure a curtailment in the use of water, measures should be taken to increase the supply, so that the entire population can have all that is desired.

As the editorial indicated, meters were certainly no closer to acceptance in 1898 than they were when Trautwine began his crusade in 1895, and the councils decided to keep filters and meters separate and tabled voting on the latter, at least for the immediate future. The mechanical filter proposed by Trautwine was also widely discussed, and the general consensus seemed to be that it should be used only if absolutely necessary. As for his experimental plant, this found little support since it was tied largely to the testing of mechanical filters.

With logic that reflected the view of many of the councilmen, the *Inquirer* commented that "There would have to be experiments with mechanical contrivances, but we do not want any mechanical contrivances. When Mr. Trautwine of-

---

[38]Ibid., 5 December 1898.

fers us a mixed plant or a mechanical plant, then we say that he is not furnishing what the city requires."[39] To be sure, the councils did not rule out as possibilities either mechanical filters or the experimental plant, but the mood of the water committee was clear at least in the fall of 1898 when on 11 October it requested the department of public works to prepare an ordinance based on slow sand filtration for the entire city. So Trautwine's report had moved things along, albeit not exactly as he had planned.

[39]*Inquirer*, 9 October 1898.

IV. A Victory for the Machine

While the city councils were discussing Trautwine's report in the autumn of 1898, politicking was already underway for the upcoming mayoral election in February. Warwick was unable to run again because the charter reforms adopted in the 1880s limited the mayor to a single four-year term. The reformers had thought this a good idea, but the change simply strengthened the power of the bosses since a mayor who could not succeed himself had little leverage over the organization, however independent he may have been. Councils could also treat the mayor with less deference toward the end of his term in office, and this happened too, as we saw in the way many councilmen treated Warwick's water proposals.

In any event the mayor's office would soon be vacant, and by the end of November, a month before the Republican party convention, the city coroner, Samuel H. Ashbridge, had established himself as a heavy favorite to win the nomination. Ashbridge was in his late 40s, vigorous and trim, with dark curly hair and a debonair waxed mustache. He lived in the 20th ward in north central Philadelphia between Girard and Susquehanna Avenues. In the 1890s this was a booming blue-collar industrial district, but it also had a sprinkling of wealthier residents who lived in the fashionable brownstones that lined north Broad Street on the western boundary of the ward. Although he did not have a north Broad address, Ashbridge ranked among the elites in the ward, having been elected in November to his fifth consecutive term as coroner. Ashbridge was also the top vote getter on the Republican ticket that fall, no doubt in part a result of all the speeches he made at patriotic rallies during the Spanish-American War.

The "splendid little war," as John Hay, the American ambassador to Britain, called it, lasted only a few weeks, from late in April to early August of 1898. Everyone expected it to be a short war after Admiral Dewey's decisive victory over the Spanish fleet in Manila Bay on 1 May. Troop recruitment was organized on a state-by-state basis as it had been during the Civil War, but only some 5,000 Pennsylvanians got a chance to sign up because the federal government asked the states for only a total of 125,000 volunteers, the war being seen primarily as a naval conflict. In the middle of May another 125,000 men were requested, but the war department moved slowly in filling the quota since it had not finished processing the first batch of recruits.[1] All this was a far cry from Civil War days when some 300,000 Pennsylvanians were in uniform, and the Union Army alone used 2.7 million troops.

For all the Philadelphians who stayed home, patriotic rallies were a way to show their support of the war. Flag raising ceremonies (usually dedicating new flag poles) were especially popular. Shortly after the war started, they were held everywhere, the most elaborate ones being at mills and factories where owners no doubt saw the opportunity to fuse patriotism with greater productivity.

Whatever the motives, the flag raisings were impressive shows. At William Wharton Jr. & Company, an iron works at 25th and Washington Avenue in South Philadelphia, for example, the festivities opened with the singing of "A Song of Liberty" by children from the neighborhood W. S. Pierce School. A chorus of Wharton employees followed them with "The Red, White and Blue," and then everyone heard "Yankee Doodle Dewey," an original song composed by one of the foremen and sung by a quartet of employees to the tune of "Yankee Doodle Dandy." Then a 15 by 25 foot American flag, bought by the employees, was pulled up a brand new 80 foot flagpole. As the flag ascended the staff, the Jefferson Band played the national anthem and the factory's

---

[1] *Inquirer,* 11, 26 May 1898.

whistles shrieked and a cannon roared a salute. When the flag reached the top of the pole, the twelve-year-old daughter of the vice-president of the company yanked a cord that opened the folds of the flag and dozens of small flags fluttered to the ground. As this was happening, six white doves were set free and flew skyward, and riflemen from the U.S. Grant Camp, No. 5, Sons of Veterans, fired a salute.[2]

Ashbridge was not one of the speakers at the Wharton Company ceremonies, but he talked at a patriotic rally the night before, and at flag raising ceremonies the next weekend at the Bethesda Presbyterian Church in Frankford and at Veterans' Hall in South Philadelphia. According to the *Public Ledger,* Ashbridge spoke at over one hundred flag raisings during the year, a good reason no doubt why he picked up the nickname "Stars and Stripes Sam."[3]

In an election year Ashbridge's patriotism was smart politics, and he attracted GOP leaders who were seeking to avoid another divisive convention like the one in 1895. The political situation was much the same as it was four years earlier, with the regulars divided into two factions. David Martin was on one side, on the other Quay and Penrose, the latter now a U.S. senator, having been chosen by the Republican legislature in 1897. State senator Israel Durham was another important member, and he watched out for the interests of Quay and Penrose while they were busy in Washington. Ever since Martin had dumped Penrose, Quay had tried to reduce Martin's influence, but he had not been very successful. In fact his efforts had more or less backfired as the district attorney's office under Graham had gone after Quay for some financial irregularities in a bank failure in Philadelphia. Quay faced an indictment in the fall of 1898, but Martin was not anxious to overplay his hand because Quay was up for re-election in 1899 and the party did not want to lose his seat to a Democrat.

Because he was not closely associated with either of the factions, Ashbridge emphasized his peace-making role in pushing his own candidacy. Ashbridge told a ward committee endorsing him that "Henceforth, not only in this ward,

[2]Ibid., 29 May 1898.
[3]*Public Ledger,* 29 December 1898.

but in every ward there will be one Republican party for all Republican citizens. After four years of warfare, old wounds are healed, battle shields are put away, and reunited Republicans can find a common enemy in the Democratic party." Ashbridge's remarks drew "prolonged applause" at the meeting since everyone knew what he was talking about, and they longed for some party concord too.[4] Martin had no favorite of his own, and he found Ashbridge suitable enough although he did not endorse him or any other hopeful. The Quay camp on the other hand wanted one of their own men, but given the popularity of Ashbridge, they were willing to go along with Ashbridge too, "in the interest of fair play and harmony," as one of the Quay leaders in South Philadelphia, select councilman William S. Vare put it.[5]

The only other serious contender for nomination was select councilman Jacob Seeds, chairman of the joint finance committee, who kicked off his own "boom" early in November at a rally at the town hall in his home ward of Germantown.[6] Seeds hoped the suburban organization leaders would back him, but they seemed happy enough with Ashbridge. Undaunted, Seeds then courted the independent reform Republicans, but even they seemed satisfied with Ashbridge and did not bother to nominate a candidate of their own. Seeds finally withdrew his name the day before the GOP convention. His decision no doubt disappointed the *Public Ledger* which preferred him, but the paper considered Ashbridge acceptable enough as did the other major dailies.

And so on 29 December, at what the *Public Ledger* called "one of the most orderly gatherings of its kind that has assembled for many years," the Republican delegates, 996 strong, met at the Academy of Music and nominated Ashbridge by acclamation, no other name even being offered to the convention. With a popular candidate and unity restored, the Republicans that day had no doubt about the election outcome, a view that was proven justified in February when after a quiet campaign, Ashbridge crushed his

[4]*Inquirer,* 1 December 1898.
[5]*Record,* 26 November 1898.
[6]*Public Ledger,* 11 November 1898.

Democratic opponent by a vote of 147,000 to 47,000 for a
new record plurality.[7]

* * *

Even before he was in office, Ashbridge found himself in
the midst of the controversy over water improvements. On
19 January a bill was introduced in the select council propos-
ing that a Quaker City Water Company supply the city with
filtered water from a new pumping station the company
would build on the Delaware River. At first glance this might
seem innocent enough, but the sponsor of the bill was councilman Lucas G. Fourier of the 28th ward, one of the insiders in the Schuylkill Valley Water Company scheme, which
made many suspicious. Moreover, the lobbyist for Quaker
City Water Company was none other than Nelson Green,
whose bribery charges had been dropped only a few weeks
earlier when the grand jury failed to find enough evidence
for an indictment.

Green was even using his old offices in the Witherspoon
Building on Walnut Street, the Quaker City Water Company
having taken them over from the Schuylkill Valley Water
Company organizers. To be sure, the new company had different stockholders and was tapping different water sources,
but the *Public Ledger* was understandably skeptical and called
the company "a new water snake," a view that was shared by
many councilmen. Bringhurst was so angry at Green's ar-
rogance that he said he would not even have the water committee consider the bill unless the other members forced him
to do so.[8]

Everyone was curious to know Ashbridge's opinion since
he was clearly going to be the city's next mayor, and he had
not really said much about water up to then in his campaign
speeches. Shortly after the Quaker City bill was introduced,
Ashbridge addressed the issue. In a letter to the Republican

---

[7]Ibid., 22 February 1899. Election figures here and elsewhere have been rounded off
to the nearest thousand.
[8]Ibid., 21 January 1899; *Inquirer*, 21 January 1899.

executive committee acknowledging his nomination, Ashbridge said that "no sale or lease of the waterworks, nor any other public franchise, will ever meet with my consent or approval."[9]

Technically the Quaker City bill was not a sale or a lease, but nearly everyone assumed Ashbridge was referring to the proposal before the councils. The *Public Ledger* wanted to be sure, and it sent a reporter to interview Ashbridge, who cleared up any ambiguity without hesitation, saying that he was against the "transfer of any part of the water system to a corporation or outside party." The new bill would do just that, he said, and he would "oppose the transfer of even the matter of furnishing or supplying water with or without a formula of a lease."[10]

With the signal strong and clear from Ashbridge, the common council introduced the following resolution at its next meeting.[11]

Whereas, There have been numerous articles published in the public press of the city, and it being the common talk among the people that our water works would be leased or sold; and Whereas, There have been bills introduced to furnish the city with filtered water by private parties or corporations; and Whereas, These Councils are of the opinion that our water works should not be leased or sold, and whatever is to be done to better our water supply should be done by the city herself, therefore be it Resolved, by the Select and Common Councils of the city of Philadelphia, That we proclaim to our citizens at large that our water works shall not be leased or sold. Resolved, That the Committee on Water be and they are hereby instructed to report back all bills with a negative recommendation, relative to the sale or lease of the water works; also the bill of the Quaker City Water Company to provide the city with a sufficient supply of filtered water, or any other private bills of like import.

The common council passed the resolution by a unanimous vote and sent it to the select council where Fourier and his friends managed to keep it from coming to a vote that day. Whether or not the select council supported the

---

[9]*Public Ledger*, 23 January 1898.
[10]Ibid., 24 January 1899.
[11]*Inquirer*, 27 January 1899.

resolution (it was later approved), Bringhurst said the Quaker City bill was "dead" so far as he was concerned. When asked by one of the bill's friends how it could be dead even before it was read or considered by a committee, Bringhurst replied it was dead because he "did not think there was enough dishonesty in the water committee to pass it."[12]

On the same day that the common council passed the resolution rebuffing the Quaker City Water Company, it also passed a bill to start moving along some of its own plans for filtration, so the "new water snake" seems to have had a positive effect so far as getting the councils to act. The bill allocated $3.2 million to build filtration plants on the Schuylkill. It was based on recommendations submitted by public works head Thompson, who had been asked by the councils to provide a proposal incorporating ideas in Trautwine's report of October 1898 and the views aired when the councils discussed the report. Thompson recommended mechanical filters for the Queen Lane pumping station and also for West Philadelphia even though the councils had preferred a plan that would use only slow sand filters. Thompson was not happy about this either, but he said there was little choice, given the large size of sand filters and the high cost of land in the Schuylkill districts.[13]

Although interest was high in the common council, the select council was in no hurry to pass the filtration bill. Or to be more precise, Fourier's followers were in no hurry. As backers of Quay and Penrose, they had never been anxious to pass anything Warwick's administration wanted. Now they had an extra reason, angry as they were that their Quaker City Water Company bill had been rejected. For weeks they kept the common council's filtration bill from coming up for a vote.

***

Fourier and his friends made the select council look es-

---
[12]Ibid.
[13]*Public Ledger*, 10 January 1899.

pecially irresponsible because the city was once again in the midst of a serious typhoid epidemic early in 1899. Typhoid cases began climbing in January and then rocketed up in February. At first health officials suspected the interceptor sewer that caused the last major outbreak in November of 1897, but the sewer was not the culprit this time, the water bureau said. No backup flow into the Schuylkill was reported, and all the manholes that leaked in the November 1897 episode had been sealed tight and showed no signs of new leakage.

The trouble this time seems to have been the chronic problem of upstream pollution, which was no doubt made worse in Philadelphia by the surging high waters that followed the melting of the snow from the great blizzard that struck the city in February. A front page editorial cartoon in the *Inquirer* entitled "Beautiful Snow Indeed" commented on the situation with bitter irony. The cartoon showed a morose William Penn standing in the midst of piles of filthy snow. One of the piles has "typhoid" written on it and Penn is saying, "Just think, in a few days that will be Schuylkill water and I shall have to drink it."[14]

The next day the *Inquirer* followed up with an editorial that blasted the councils.[15]

There were thirty-eight deaths from typhoid fever in this city last week, and for each of the deaths the men who sit in council chambers and waste their time in a sterile and illusory debate of a question, every phase of which has been worn threadbare by interminable discussion, are morally responsible. There were 287 new cases of typhoid fever in this city last week, and for each of those cases the councilmen who, whether from incompetence or indifference, or because of reasons still more reprehensible, persist in their refusal or their failure—it makes no difference which—to take any definitive action in the matter of such vital consequence to the community, are accountable to their constituents. . . . Even in New York, where the prevailing conditions of life are far less favorable to health than they are in Philadelphia, the mortality from typhoid has, since the installation of the new Croton River aqueduct, been reduced to proportions quite inconsiderable.

---

[14]*Inquirer,* 19 February 1899.
[15]Ibid., 20 February 1899.

Thus in one week last month, among a population of over three million, only fourteen cases and six deaths were reported. Compare that with our thirty-eight deaths and 287 cases! When the reason for the terrible discrepancy is so well known, where there is such an absolute agreement as to the remedy necessary to be applied, is it not monstrous that our councilmen continue to talk, talk, talk and do nothing! How can they rest easy, how can they sleep at night, and look their fellow citizens in the face in the daytime, with this awful load of responsibility resting upon them? They must, one would think, have the skin of a rhinoceros and the consciences so calloused as to be proof against any impression.

As we have seen, not all the councilmen were as irresponsible as the *Inquirer* claimed, but it was also true that when the editorial appeared on 20 February, the select council seemed to be a long way from approving the filtration bill passed by the common council on 26 January. All hopes of getting the bill through the upper chamber were largely in the hands of the co-chairman of the water committee, select councilman Robert Bringhurst of the 9th ward in Center City. A big man with pince-nez glasses, black hair and a mustache and goatee, Bringhurst had a forceful personality to match his imposing mien. Bringhurst was a respected and successful businessman who was the head of a prominent funeral home still in business today. His occupation must have made him a natural butt for jokes, so it is little wonder that he was sensitive about the water issue. He was also livid with Fourier and his friends for hurting the reputation of all the responsible men in the councils. "Nowadays as I walk along the street, and hear remarks made that I am a councilman," he remarked ruefully, "I do not know whether to run or simply dodge."[16]

However conscientious he may have been, it should be noted that Bringhurst dragged his own feet for a while after the common council had approved the filtration bill. Bringhurst had not been happy about its provisions for mechanical filters at the two pumping stations on the Schuylkill. He wanted instead a massive slow sand filtration plant on the Delaware, along the lines of something that public works

---

[16]Ibid., 10 March 1899.

head Thompson had talked to the councils about in a report they received on 9 January 1899. Thompson said the city's long range plan should include a new filtration plant on the Delaware River in the far northeast section of the city where the river was cleanest. Everyone recognized that the Delaware was a much better source than the Schuylkill, and it made sense to build a big new pumping station there before the city ran into serious water shortages.

Bringhurst had managed to get this idea approved in the select council on 26 January, and for a week or so he seemed to prefer that bill to the common council's bill for the Schuylkill River plants. But the cost of a large filtration plant on the Delaware would far exceed the $3.3 million available through the loan bill, and early in February Bringhurst changed his mind, no doubt realizing that the city had to start somewhere—and soon, given the mounting death toll. "The people want them," he said in announcing that he would push for mechanical filtration plants on the Schuylkill as a first step, his own opinions notwithstanding.[17]

Early in March Bringhurst and like-minded colleagues, who comprised the majority in the select council, finally overcame Fourier's postponement tactics and scheduled a vote for 9 March. When the select council met that day, Bringhurst pointed out that the bill was simply to authorize the director of public works to advertise bids that would afterward have to be approved by the councils. Noting that there had been a wide difference among the experts as to what the total costs would be for all the improvements, Bringhurst said, "We do not know which is right, and the object of this ordinance is to enable us to find out what can be done. Every member who is sincere and honest in his desire to settle the water problem will vote for it. It brings to this Council the information of the world."[18]

Fourier was less interested in getting information than in pointing out the ordinance's failings. The proposal in the bill would not filter the water for a tenth of the city, he said. One of his friends, William Vare, the South Philadelphia politician who was also a Quay man, picked up this point and

---

[17]Ibid., 8 February 1899.
[18]Ibid., 10 March 1899.

complained that the bill would not help his constituents. All this was true but also irrelevant since the councilmen knew they did not have enough money in the loan bill to filter the entire city.

Another Quay man, Joseph Nobre of the 2nd ward in south Philadelphia, urged the council to "go slow." He asked, "What are the people going to get if this bill passed? Is filtered water going to put out a fire or flush the sewer any better than unfiltered water? I'm told there is a dredger up the river that is used whenever necessary to stir up the mud and make the people think the water is bad. I haven't seen it, but I've been told it is there. I am firmly convinced that filtration is no good. Why, you know that there are plenty of times throughout the year when the water is just as good as anyone wants to drink who doesn't drink beer." Views on filtration were aired for two hours, with supporters of the bill getting some time on the floor too, before voting took place. The bill was approved 18-10, but it was three votes short of the two-thirds majority needed for funding ordinances. Fortunately for the filtration backers the measure was not dead, thanks to widespread protest after the vote, and another vote was scheduled for 23 March.

At this stage the question everyone was asking was what mayor-elect Ashbridge planned to do. He had not said anything against the filtration bill, but he had not said anything for it either. In fact he was not in the city at all for over two weeks, having left on 22 February for a vacation in Florida and Cuba. When he returned on 10 March, it was clear that Ashbridge was hoping that no legislation would be passed until he took office in mid-April. To be sure, he did not say or do anything indiscreet; rather he sought to get his way by asking everyone to wait a little.

On 18 March, the day after the select council had officially revived the bill, Ashbridge met with Bringhurst in what seemed an attempt at coopting the chairman of the water committee. Flattered by the attention and the interest of the mayor-elect in his work, Bringhurst told the press he was impressed by Ashbridge's grasp of water matters. Bringhurst did not say he was not going to push for passage of the filtration bill at the next meeting of the select council, but it was also obvious that he would not be overly concerned if the bill did not pass, Ashbridge having promised that he would have a bill of his own ready within a few weeks after he was in office.[19]

Ashbridge used much the same strategy with community groups. Unable to attend a water meeting in Germantown on 22 March, Ashbridge sent a letter saying that he was devoting nearly all his time to the water issue and asked that his administration be given "a fair and reasonable time" to introduce its proposals. The details would be worked out shortly—within a couple of weeks in fact. He could not be more specific, he said, because "It would be unfair to express my plans in advance of sending them to City Councils."[20]

The mayor-elect's lobbying for delay notwithstanding, the councils were still considering the current filtration bill, and the day before the second vote was to be taken, the Citizens Emergency Committee met at the Board of Trade offices in the Bourse building near Independence Hall. Frank Firth, the president of the City Organizations' Filtration Committee, said he was willing to wait for Ashbridge, resigned as he was to the fact that nothing apparently was going to happen while Warwick was still in office. Firth said the current situation in the councils was hopeless because the Quay people would not pass anything Warwick wanted. Ashbridge on the other hand was not allied to either faction, and the chances of success would be greater with him in office. Dr. H.C. Woods agreed with Firth, saying

It is to Mayor Ashbridge we should look in the midst of this chaos and death and not the Councils. Let us appoint a committee to wait upon the Mayor. Then there will be the possibility of achieving something. If the Mayor fails us, then it will be time for a public meeting.[21]

George Woodward, a Germantown physician, disagreed with the "wait and see" attitude and recommended a demonstration at City Hall. In his view, the councils will do nothing unless they are forced to. "If we could have 100,000 people

---

[19]Ibid., 18 March 1899.
[20]*Public Ledger*, 23 March 1899.
[21]*Inquirer*, 23 March 1899.

at the City Hall," he said, "the councils would shake in their boots."[22] He got applause for his suggestion, but the committee decided instead to send a delegation to attend the select council meeting the next day when the vote would be taken. This idea was strongly supported by common councilman Herman Loeb of the 32nd ward in West Philadelphia. He thought the select council would pass the bill, but he also thought their presence in the chamber would have "a good effect."[23]

And so the stage was set for the second vote on the filtration bill. The day started unpropitiously for the Citizens Emergency Committee when their members arrived, some twenty-five in number, at the council chambers only to be denied entrance by the doorkeepers. They could go to the spectators' gallery, the doorkeepers said, but no one except council members was permitted on the floor during sessions. Apparently no one had alerted the doorkeepers, or even members of the select council for that matter, because the delegation was led into the clerk's office where they had to wait for over an hour while the select council decided what to do. By then the spectators' gallery was packed so that the floor of the chamber appeared to be the only place they could go, whether the councilmen wanted them there or not.

Bringhurst asked for the suspension of rule 34, which forbade visitors on the floor during sessions. This would give the Citizens Emergency Committee "the privilege" of attending, he said, without of course taking any part in the proceedings. "They are reputable gentlemen, and are here in the interest that is dear to the heart of every citizen." Select councilman Nobre then got up and said, "I have no objection to citizens being here, but it occurs to me that this is a little in the line of sharp practice. I do not think there is a member here who could not bring seventy five people from his ward if he wished. I have only one objection to the admission of this committee. I hope there will be no lobbying." Bringhurst replied testily,

---

[22]*Public Ledger*, 23 March 1899.
[23]Ibid.

These gentlemen came here as a representative body and ask that they be allowed the privilege of the floor. This is no request of mine, but the citizens propose to ask by their silent presence that this water question be settled promptly. It is a good sign when these men lay aside their business for an afternoon and make efforts to do away with a desperate nuisance.

Unimpressed and getting angry himself, Nobre replied, "I am just as eager as the gentleman from the Ninth ward to get good water, but I do not think it is decent or fair to tie the incoming mayor for four years with any legislation we may pass. I have no interest in any scheme or any plan excepting to furnish the people with good water. I have no interest in appropriating over $3 million just to furnish a small section of the people with filtered water. I am not in favor of this appropriation, and I will not allow any man to stand up and by insinuation throw rocks at my reputation. I am ready at the proper time to vote for any plan that will give the entire city pure water."[24]

After that opening exchange, things quieted down, and the council approved the admission of the committee members, who stood along the wall of the chambers since there were no empty seats on the floor. Bringhurst tried to be as persuasive as possible when he opened the discussion on the bill. "It needs no argument to convince the minds of the members that the water supplied today is unfit for use," he said. "The quality is wrong. It doesn't require much time to settle this question. We are told that typhoid is flourishing at an extravagant rate in this city, and it is time that something is done. Let's lay aside all politics and all nonsense. In passing this ordinance you are doing no harm, furthering no scheme."

Councilman Clay, who had been outspoken in his criticism of the private water company schemes, backed Bringhurst. Admitting that the funds in the loan bill could not filter the entire city, Clay pointed out that "It was the most money we have available, and the reputation of our city calls upon us to make this appropriation. I believe the gentleman who has

---

[24]*Inquirer,* 24 March 1899.

been elected mayor is prompted by sincere motives when he says he will give his undivided attention to the settlement of the water question, and if so, what better way can we make known to him our ideas than to put at his disposal the sum of $3.2 million toward helping him to solve the problem?"[25]

Despite the logic, Clay's speech had no effect on the opponents of the bill. As Fourier and others joined Nobre in attacking it in long-winded speeches, members of the Citizens Emergency Committee saw what was happening, and in groups of twos and threes they began drifting off to the doors and leaving the chamber. By the time the vote was taken at 6:30 p.m. only a half dozen remained. Once again the bill got a majority—this time the vote was 24-13 because more members were present—but the figures fell three votes short of the two-thirds necessary. Down a second time, the bill was finished so far as that session of the councils was concerned.

The reformers of course were disappointed, as they had been when the same thing happened earlier in the month. At that time Bringhurst had criticized the mayor for not helping more, but there was little persuading that Warwick could do, as unpopular as he was with the Quay and Penrose people and a "lame duck" mayor who would soon be out of office. It must have been an especially frustrating time for Warwick. At a Philadelphia County Medical Society dinner in January the mayor was scheduled to give an address on "The Doctor's Duty to the New Philadelphia," but he was unable to attend. The audience laughed when Vice President Dr. Solomon Solis-Cohen said he was disappointed because he had intended to ask the mayor when the city would get better water than "the bacteriological mixture" now supplied by the water bureau.

Applause for Warwick followed, however, when Solis-Cohen added, "So far as Mayor Warwick is concerned, he has done his share in trying to give us something else." The physicians at least recognized that the mayor was not responsible for the delays.[26] Solis-Cohen in fact had been one of several prominent physicians Warwick had appointed to a

[25]Ibid.
[26]*Public Ledger*, 17 January 1899.

committee to advise him on the water problem. Warwick had always shown a genuine interest in public health, backing, for example, the successful efforts of Philadelphians to get the American Public Health Association to hold its 25th anniversary meeting in the city in October of 1897.

Bringhurst also criticized Trautwine, and the head of the water bureau was more culpable in the sense that he refused to compromise and kept on talking about the need for his experimental station even after the idea had been rejected by the councils. Worse still, Trautwine never gave up his crusade for water meters, which made him seem very naive indeed in the eyes of the councilmen who were unwilling to risk their seats to push that controversial issue with the voters.

In fairness to Trautwine, there seemed to be some truth in his contention that waste contributed to the severity of the recent outbreak of typhoid. Water usually stayed a few days in reservoirs where sedimentation made it a bit safer, but for a few days in January of 1899 the water demand was so high in some districts served by the Queen Lane pumping station that the water spent little more than an hour in the reservoir before going into the distributing mains. To keep up the supply, the water bureau had also pumped water directly from the Spring Garden pumping station to some houses in the 15th and 29th wards that were normally served by the Queen Lane reservoir. This meant in effect raw water was going into those houses.

In any event, the number of typhoid cases among residents getting water from Queen Lane and Spring Garden was much higher than elsewhere. In Trautwine's view, meters would have reduced unnecessary consumption, which in turn would have kept more water in the reservoirs for longer periods of time and therefore increased the benefits of the sedimentation. All this made sense, but the logic of Trautwine's reasoning was lost on nearly everyone including Bringhurst who felt that filtration should come first, not water meters.

The head of the bacteriology department in the board of health, Dr. Alexander C. Abbott, was also surprisingly inept in selling filtration to the public. In an interview that ap-

peared in the *Public Ledger* on 25 February, Abbott said that
no filter, not even one made of fine grained porcelain, could
prevent typhoid bacilli from passing through, especially if
the water passed through under pressure as it would at a
pumping station. This was quite true, but filters did not have
to be one hundred percent effective in order to save lives, as
Abbott well knew. He could have emphasized the positive
side of the filtration in his interview. Instead he said the only
certain way to kill typhoid bacilli was to boil the water. This
was also true, but to the layman it made it sound as though
filtration was worthless.

As for the "typhoid thirteen," as the *Public Ledger* dubbed
the select councilmen who killed the bill, some opposition
was almost inevitable, given the limited number of wards
receiving filtered water. Several of the councilmen who
voted "no" were from South Philadelphia, which was not
getting any filtered water from the bill. The Northeast was
another section that would not benefit, and two of the three
councilmen from wards there were also "no" voters. Of the
remaining five "no" voters, three came from select councilmen representing Center City wards which would also not
have gotten any better water. The other "no" voters were
Fourier and councilman Hamilton W. Sherlock who repre-
sented districts in North Philadelphia that would have bene-
fited directly from a filtering station at Queen Lane. It is
hard to imagine how these two could have justified their vote
to their constituents, but the other eleven might have gotten
away with it, given some fast talking. To be sure, we see
exceptions in some of the "yes" votes, Bringhurst and two
other Center City councilmen supporting the measure that
would not directly benefit their wards, but on the whole
there is a fairly strong correlation in the voting.

Various variables notwithstanding, it does appear that the
"typhoid thirteen" were simply out to kill the bill in their
personal vendetta against Mayor Warwick and his mentor,
David Martin. Not one of the thirteen was a Martin man,
and none had been a Warwick backer during the nomination
controversy in 1895. They had opposed him for four years,
and their knockout blow to the water bill in the last days of

his administration, though not very sportsmanlike, was consistent with their earlier attitude.

***

Whatever the reasons for the defeat of the bill, the attention was now on Ashbridge, who took office early in April. The water problem was the most important issue facing the city, he said in his inaugural address to the councils. Three days later he presented his ideas in more detail. The loan money would not be enough to improve the entire system, but the city had an extra $14 million credit within its current debt limit, or more than enough for bonds to fund the complete project. Before he recommended anything specific, Ashbridge wanted some experts to take another look at the water system and provide a report by early September when the councils would be back from their summer recess.[27] The study meant more delay of course, but by April the typhoid epidemic had ended and so had the crisis mentality. A few more months would not matter if the matter was finally settled, and the councils approved the mayor's proposal.

Ashbridge named to the commission Rudolph Hering of New York, Samuel M. Gray of Providence, and Joseph M. Wilson of Philadelphia, all respected engineers. Ashbridge asked them to consider three questions. "What is necessary for the immediate betterment of our water system? If the remedy be filtration, what is the best method?" and "In what direction is it most desirable to extend our present supply, so that for years to come the water problem may not give anxiety to our people?" The commissioners looked at all the old reports, studied the published results of experiments on filtration in Providence, Louisville, Cincinnati, and Pittsburgh, and visited filtration plants in Wilmington, Poughkeepsie, and Albany as well as a sewerage plant in Allentown. They inspected all the city's pumping stations and reservoirs,

---

[27]*Inquirer*, 4, 7 April 1899.

and they took trips to see the watersheds of the Schuylkill and Delaware Rivers, as well as those of Perkiomen and Lehigh. So a busy summer.

Their report did not have any surprises. Regardless of the source of the city's water, a filtration system was necessary to insure against chance contamination. They recommended the continued use of the Schuylkill and Delaware Rivers. Water from upcountry sources might be preferable but the great cost of building aqueducts and upcountry reservoirs made that option very expensive and really unnecessary since filtration would provide safe water, and the Schuylkill and Delaware were capable of meeting the city's needs for the foreseeable future.[28]

Ashbridge later admitted he favored the idea of taking water from an upcountry source, but he was quite willing to go along with the experts' recommendations, especially since their estimates fell within the current borrowing capacity. The councils also accepted the report, and on 29 September they approved Ashbridge's request for a $12 million bond issue, to supplement the funds already approved for filtration. At a referendum on 3 November, the spending was approved without any controversy. Ashbridge sent to the councils on 15 November five ordinances totaling $15.2 million ($12 million approved in the recent referendum and $3.2 from the earlier one) which would get the actual construction underway. The $3.2 million was earmarked for filtration plants on the Schuylkill. This was similar to the project held up earlier in the year (slow sand filters would be installed this time). The rest of the money went for other filtration plants and improvements to pumping stations, pipelines, and the like. The ordinances were favorably received, approved by the water committee, and then passed easily by both councils in January of 1900. And so water reform, controversial for so long, quietly became a reality.

While approval was expected, the degree to which the councils acceded to mayoral control over the construction was quite surprising, considering the way the councils had guarded their prerogatives with Warwick. The issue arose at

[28]First Annual Message of Samuel H. Ashbridge in Board of Health, *Annual Report* (1899), xv-xvii.

a meeting of the water committee early in January when an amendment had been offered to give the councils final approval of project specifications and costs. All the water bills during Warwick's term had been worded this way, so the idea behind the amendment was neither new, nor controversial, but select councilman Clay protested.

"The councils are merely agents of the people," Clay said, and since the people had approved the loan, authority should be given to the mayor to carry out the program.[29] This was nonsense, another councilman said, who pointed out to Clay that the vote of the people gave the council the authority to oversee appropriations. "The people have not relieved councils from their responsibility in this matter or given them any binding instructions." Another councilman added that if the mayor had unlimited control of expenditures, the councils "might as well be abolished."[30]

The truth was somewhere in the middle. Clay was right that the charter reforms in the 1880s intended to strengthen the mayor's office, but it was also true that the councils could monitor appropriations closely if they so chose, as they did with the water bills that Warwick's administration offered. On the other hand, as Bringhurst pointed out during the debate, the councils had not required an item-by-item review of all the public works projects they had approved when Warwick was in office. Ashbridge's new director of public works, William C. Haddock, was highly regarded and able to do the job without the councils looking over his shoulder, Bringhurst implied, praising Haddock's honesty with the remark that "We have never heard of any dirt sticking to his clothes."[31] Bringhurst, however, was unable to convince the majority of the committee, who voted 13-9 for council control.

A week later when the first of the water bills came to the full chambers for a final vote, the councils dropped the amendment without any fight.[32] It is not exactly clear why there was such a quick change of view. To be sure, the press

---

[29]*Inquirer,* 5 January 1899.
[30]Ibid.
[31]Ibid.
[32]*Inquirer,* 12 January 1899.

had criticized the amendment, with views ranging from the *Public Ledger*'s mild remark that it was "unnecessary" to the *Inquirer*'s opinion that wayward members of the water committee who had voted for the amendment were interested only in keeping their fingers in "The Fifteen Million Dollar Water Pie."[33] Pressure from the press may have helped, but the councils may also have felt that the amendment was not necessary. They trusted the mayor, and he promised to work closely with them on all phases of the water improvements.

Whatever the reasons he got his way, Ashbridge must be given high marks for his skill and speed in handling the water issue. In ten months he had presented his program and hired consultants who delivered on time a report that met with council approval; his loan legislation was accepted by the councils and voters, and Ashbridge had pushed the ordinances that actually got the work underway, winning a free hand to oversee all the details as well. His move for a commission was especially deft since it seemed to help reach consensus on the best way to settle the water question. As noted earlier, there was nothing really new in the report, the experts having confirmed earlier findings, but this of course was just why the report was so effective, providing as it did the imprimatur of respected authorities for ideas that were already gaining widespread support.

Skillful as Ashbridge may have been in getting filtration approved and underway, he also owed much of his success simply to his being a popular regular who got along with the various party factions. It is unlikely that the councils would have been so cooperative if Warwick had still been in office. At the same time it is also unlikely that the councils could have procrastinated much longer, given the public furor and the solid evidence that filtration worked in combatting typhoid. In any event, career machine politician that he was, Ashbridge perhaps was just the right sort of mayor to coax filtration through councils dominated by machine politicians.

As for Trautwine, Ashbridge kept him on as chief of the water bureau, primarily because the outside experts working

---

[33]*Public Ledger*, 10 January 1899; *Inquirer*, 7 January 1899.

on the commission felt he would be useful to have around
when they prepared their report. Apparently Trautwine was
a help in the busy summer of 1899 when the work was done,
but he was not happy with the final report because he still
felt water meters should be installed before moving ahead
with filtration, in order to reduce overall costs by reducing
consumption. Ashbridge differed with Trautwine on this issue, so it is not surprising that Trautwine resigned in
November shortly after the voters approved the filtration
plan.

Despite their differences, Ashbridge shared many of
Trautwine's concerns about water waste. The first bill in fact
that Ashbridge introduced was for new buildings to have
flush toilets with valves that shut off the water when the tank
was refilled, and it was approved by the councils. A bill for
meters in the fall of 1899 was also introduced before Trautwine resigned, but the councils still opposed the idea. Ashbridge wisely avoided pushing for approval since it could
have jeopardized the filtration bills. Ashbridge wanted results, not quixotic crusades, and his attitude seemed more
responsible than Trautwine's, given the deaths involved in
more delays. In any case, Ashbridge picked Frank L. Hand,
a respected water bureau veteran, to be the new chief, so the
caliber of the leadership stayed high.

V. Construction and More Controversy

Clinton Rogers Woodruff was a lawyer and a reformer who was not much involved in the water story aside from helping in the bribery investigation in 1898. Woodruff was more interested in keeping an eye on voter fraud in municipal elections, and he later served for many years as president of the city's voter registration board. He was also secretary and then counsel of the Philadelphia Municipal League in the 1890s and early 1900s; and secretary of the National Municipal League, and editor of the proceedings of the National Conference for Good City Government. In this latter role in particular Woodruff became regarded as the reform authority on Philadelphia.

In November of 1899 Woodruff published an article entitled "Philadelphia's Water: A Story of Municipal Procrastination," in the genteel *Forum*. Although he seemed to prefer an upstream aqueduct solution, Woodruff was happy that something was finally done. With little confidence in the machine, however, he cautioned that "From past experience we are no means out of danger," since "the money had to be formally appropriated, the contracts given, and the work completed."[1] Woodruff's worries would be justified, but at least the project got off to a good start.

Work began first on the Lower Roxborough filtration plant in Northwest Philadelphia. Five filter beds were built there, each a little more than a half acre in size and each capable of filtering 1.6 million gallons of Schuylkill River

---

[1]*Forum* 28 (November 1899), 314. Biographical material from sketch in *Who's Who in Pennsylvania* (Chicago, 1939), 977.

water daily.[2] The filters were made of concrete, and each could be shut down separately for cleaning. The beds were built into the ground and covered with flat roofs, to prevent the water from freezing and to reduce air pollution. They were designed with plenty of overhead space inside because workmen had to get in them regularly to drain and clean the filters. The ceilings were twenty feet high supported by arched pillars at fourteen foot intervals. In one construction photograph an empty filter looks almost like a gallery in a medieval cathedral, pier after pier of graceful columns going off in every direction and soft sunlight streaming down through ventilator holes high overhead.[3]

A similar plant was built at Upper Roxborough to serve Chestnut Hill, Mt. Airy, and parts of Germantown. The two Roxborough plants went into operation in 1903. Another plant at Belmont Avenue near City Avenue in West Philadelphia began filtering water the following year. The plants were operating before all their filter beds were completed, in order to provide safer water as soon as possible. In 1905, the first year of filtration, the typhoid rate dropped an average of ninety percent in the wards getting filtered water, and the case per 100,000 per week in the those wards was 0.53 compared to the city-wide average of 5.53 cases.[4]

In 1906 a serious outbreak of typhoid struck again in unfiltered districts, with a death toll that year of 1,063, up from 684 in 1905. This was the worst annual death toll from typhoid since the city began keeping records on the disease in 1861, and it underscored the need to get the entire system in operation as soon as possible.[5] The biggest of the filtration plants was then under construction at Torresdale on the Delaware River, a few miles north of Frankford above the mouth of Pennypack Creek. Fifty filters, forty-eight acres in area, would have a filtering capacity of over 200 million

---

[2]Bureau of Water, *Annual Report* (1901), 235 ff.
[3]Ibid., opposite 238.
[4]Bureau of Filtration *Annual Report* (1906), table following page 222.
[5]Warner in *Private City* cites the 1906 epidemic as an example of how late Philadelphia was still having major problems, but he does not mention the filtration work already underway. He leaves the impression that water reform came after 1906 by saying "In 1910-1911 filters and chlorine brought relief from these recurrent epidemics" (109).

gallons daily. This was more than the combined total of a dozen filtering plants then serving London and made Torresdale the largest single plant in the world at the time. Unfortunately a political controversy in 1905 temporarily stopped construction. Critics claimed this contributed to the high death toll in the typhoid epidemic the following year, but this is not accurate because the rest of the system was not ready even if the conduit had been completed. In any event, this was an important episode in the filtration story, and it is worth examining in some detail.

The mayor in 1905 was John Weaver, a GOP regular and a former district attorney who had the support of both the machine and reformers. By that time David Martin had been eased out of leadership of the local organization, and the new head was Israel Durham, the backer of the old Quay and Penrose clique. (Quay died in 1904, and Penrose was now the leader in Washington.) While respectable enough, Weaver was not a Warwick and after his election in 1903, the machine began to take Weaver for granted—to his growing dismay.[6] In May of 1905 when regulars in the councils, acting on Durham's orders, approved a controversial gas ordinance that Weaver opposed, the mayor retaliated by firing two top appointees who were Durham men: the head of public safety and the head of public works. Weaver then launched investigations into the bureaus, in hopes of finding something that would make his actions look like more than political pique—and to hold on to the support of reformers who were cheering him. (The councils also dropped the gas ordinance after Weaver vetoed it.)

And so, almost inevitably, the filtration project was drawn into the controversy. Created as a separate unit from the water bureau in 1902, the bureau of filtration oversaw the construction work. The head was John Wilmuth Hill, who came from Cincinnati in 1900. He was an authority on typhoid problems and regarded as one of the country's leading engineers in the field of public health. Hill had worked hard

---

[6]As an indication of how lopsided party strengths were in those years, Weaver crushed his Democratic opponent in the mayoral election by a 169,000 to 33,000 vote, a plurality that broke the previous record set by Ashbridge in 1899. *Inquirer*, 19 February 1903.

in getting filtration underway, and when fishing expeditions began in his bureau, he lost patience with Philadelphia politics and resigned.

To investigate Hill's work, Weaver brought in Donald Maclennan, an engineer who had been in charge of the building of the filtration plant in Washington, D.C., and Cassius Gillette, an army engineer who had some experience in investigations of this kind, having recently helped to prepare charges for fraud involving harbor improvements in Savannah, Georgia. Weaver also asked William Parsons, a consulting engineer on the Panama Canal project which was then underway. Parsons declined to serve, blaming the press of other business, a decision critics of Weaver interpreted as an indication that Parsons had no desire to get involved in what seemed a political vendetta.

A report prepared by Maclennan and Gillette was released just before the fall elections in November, a move which gave some credence to the belief in its political inspiration. It said the filtration project had wasted six million dollars, but its authors offered no explanation as to how they had reached the sum.[7] Brothers John and Daniel McNichol, both friendly with Durnham, held the largest number of contracts, but they denied any charge of excessive profits. On ten contracts they had completed, for which they received total payments of $3.9 million, the McNichols claimed they barely made money, winding up with only a 9 percent profit on the contracts let, a figure below the 20 percent that Gillette and Maclennan said was an acceptable margin of profit.

Undaunted, Weaver brought John Hill to trial on several counts of irregularities in handling contracts. All the charges were dismissed for lack of evidence against Hill, who was defended by George Graham, the respected district attorney of the Warwick years. Among the major daily papers, the *Inquirer* was the only one openly sympathetic to Hill, no doubt because it was the only paper supporting the regular organization in the split between Durnham and Weaver. The *Ledger, Bulletin,* and *Record* grudgingly agreed that Hill was

---

[7] The complete report is reprinted in the Appendix to the *Journal of the Select Council* (5 October 1905-29 March 1906), 47-77. The report was released on 29 October 1905.

innocent of the charges, but they preferred to consider him guilty anyway, apparently on the grounds that he let contracts to a firm friendly with the organization.

The report submitted by the engineers in the fall of 1905 also seemed to influence the reform press against Hill. The *Bulletin* said, for example, that "Mr. Hill has been acquitted because of a failure to establish a case against him, and he deserves the full benefit of the acquittal in the public estimate of his character. But what in the meanwhile is to become of the Gillette report, with its extraordinary charges against the entire filtration work, together with the scandal of the six million dollars loss which Gillette has alleged?"[8] Doubts like this kept the filtration project under a cloud, the view in reform circles persisting that it was akin in spirit to Tweed's court house jobbery. This seems unfair, and it might be useful to look closely at the Torresdale project, or more precisely the Torresdale conduit, because this was another McNichol contract and the focal point of the controversy.

The Torresdale conduit was a two and one-half mile long tunnel made of brick, ten feet, seven inches in diameter and one hundred feet deep that ran from the Torresdale filtration station to Lardner's Point in Frankford where the water was distributed to the rest of the city. The original plans suggested by the board of experts in 1899 had called for four parallel iron pipelines, each one foot in diameter for this section. When the city decided to increase the filtration capacity of Torresdale from 200,000 to 300,000 gallons daily (so that more of its water would be from the cleaner Delaware), the plan had to be re-evaluated.

The cost of a twelve-pipe system that would be needed to carry the increased load was estimated at nearly $3.3 million. A brick conduit would cost $2 million less, so Hill opted for the big tunnel.[9] Given the differences in cost, it is not surprising that the mayor and councils concurred, nor was there any grumbling about the decision once the work was underway. If anything, the conduit was quite popular because in addition to the savings involved, it was a sophisti-

[8]*Bulletin*, 13 January 1906.
[9]Bureau of Filtration, *Annual Report* (1904), 244-245.

cated project that gave the city a good deal of favorable publicity.

The Torresdale conduit operated on a vacuum principle, and in engineering circles it was called an inverted syphon. The distributing pumps at Lardner's Point pulled water into the conduit at the Torresdale end, so that in effect the system needed only one set of pumps. A single conduit also greatly reduced water friction compared to conventional pipelines and made it easier to move great volumes of water through quickly. While streamlined in engineering principles and theory, the job turned out to be a great deal more difficult than expected.

Rock deposits in some sections required heavy blasting and extremely slow going. With the route of the conduit close to the Delaware River and well below water level, large amounts of water also leaked into the tunnel during the digging. Even after the conduit was completed, some leakage continued, mostly of the weeping variety through the brickwork, but this was not considered serious because the water pressure inside would be greater than outside when the conduit was in service, so that whatever leakage took place, it would be filtered water going out, not contaminated water coming in.[10]

Even though there were no real health risks, Hill did not take the leakage problem lightly. After the contractors were finished in April of 1904, he carefully monitored the amount of water in the empty conduit by dropping measuring devices down the shafts. When he found leakage worse than expected, he ordered the contractors to bring in pumping equipment and empty the conduit. Inspectors found that two sumps had not been closed, which accounted for most of the leakage. The McNichol brothers had to make good on the faulty work. Doing it right the second time cost them some $22,000 because bringing back pumping equipment and emptying the conduit took several weeks and hundreds of manhours to complete. "Haste makes waste," Hill said, and it turned out to be expensive too.[11]

---

[10] Ibid., 273.
[11] Ibid., 255.

Some weeping continued through the brickwork as it was expected to do, but it was not significant. Hill told a meeting of engineers in February of 1905 that he could have made the conduit watertight by encircling it with an iron casing. But the estimated costs were so high that he considered it a foolish expenditure since there was no real health benefit, and the amount of filtered water that would be lost through leakage was not enough to make the iron casing cost-effective. The consensus among the engineers at the meeting was that Hill did the right thing by rejecting the iron casing idea.[12]

And so the Torresdale conduit story ended, or so it seemed, until the spring and summer of 1905 when the political fireworks began, and Hill resigned. In December the conduit was not yet in use because the rest of the Torresdale system was still under construction. Still acting as an investigator for Weaver (and soon to be appointed head of the filtration bureau), Gillette made an inspection tour and found some leakage. It seemed to be no more than Hill expected when the conduit was empty and water pressure greater on the outside. But soon after Gillette ordered extensive patching repairs, claiming that the construction was faulty.[13]

How could Gillette have done this after this sort of leakage was recognized among engineers as not only harmless but inevitable under nearly all conditions when a conduit was empty? The question is difficult to answer with any degree of certainty, but his decision certainly reflects poorly on his engineering ability if he really did think there was a problem.

On the other hand, Gillette may well have felt forced to do something as a political move to support Weaver, and the leaks provided him with dramatic "proof" of faulty workmanship. Whatever his reasons, Gillette remained adamant that the conduit was faulty despite the contrary testimony of experts at Hill's trial. In 1907 the new mayor, another Re-

[12]Hill, "The Torresdale Conduit," *Proceedings of the Engineers' Club of Philadelphia* 22 (June 1905): 129-183 (paper); 183-189 (discussion). Parts of this paper are included in the *Annual Report* (1904) of the Bureau of Filtration.
[13]*Inquirer* 31 December 1905; Fourth Annual Message of John Weaver in Bureau of Water, *Annual Report* (1906), lix-lvi.

publican regular John E. Reyburn, fired Gillette and appointed one of Hill's former assistants to complete the filtration project. In his annual report for 1907 the new head called the extra work unnecessary and tartly noted that Gillette's bills had run to $184,301.27.[14]

Gillette could not have gone ahead unless a few other engineers agreed with him. Influential support came from none other than our erstwhile water bureau chief, John Trautwine. Trautwine did not openly attack Hill or play any role in the politics of the Weaver administration, but his disapproval of Hill's conduit was well known and no doubt gave more respectability to Gillette's claims than they would have received otherwise. Why Trautwine wound up in Gillette's camp is not altogether clear, but at least some guesses can be made. Trautwine had worked closely with the board of experts, so that in many respects Hill was changing Trautwine's plans too, and professional pique may have been at the root of Trautwine's complaints about the conduit.

But to give him his due, Trautwine also seemed to have some honest doubts about the structural integrity of the conduit. At the meeting of the Engineers Club in 1905 when Hill read his paper, Trautwine asked him if the blasting in parts of the conduit during construction could have cracked the outer walls and caused the leaking problem. Hill described the precautions taken and said there was no evidence whatsoever that the blasting was at fault. Trautwine did not seem entirely convinced, and when the investigation got underway later in the year, he may have felt that Gillette's extra cement was really going to do something useful.[15]

Less easily explained away as an honest difference of opinion were Trautwine's remarks to a group of visiting engineers in Philadelphia in 1908. In a paper he read on the history of the water works from its origins to the present, Trautwine repeated Gillette's claim that some six million dollars had been wasted in the filtration project.[16] Given the lack of evidence, it seems a bit irresponsible on Trautwine's

[14]Bureau of Water, *Annual Report* (1907), 48.
[15]Hill, "The Torresdale Conduit," 183-186.
[16]Trautwine, "A Glance at the Water Supply of Philadelphia," *Journal of the New England Water Works Association,* 22 (1908), 439.

part, but right down to the end he remained faithful to his belief in meters and water economy. In Trautwine's view Philadelphians should have been able to make do with a system that supplied 200 million gallons of filtered water, as the report of 1899 recommended. Given this outlook, Trautwine no doubt felt the bigger system was wasteful, whether or not there was any actual graft involved.

In any event, the controversy died out, and the Torresdale work resumed. The plant went into service in stages with the first pipefuls of filtered water leaving on 15 July 1907 for neighborhoods east of Germantown Avenue and north of Lehigh Avenue, a district that included most of the northeast section of the city. As more filters at Torresdale went into service, the city's filtered water supply rose steadily, to 53 percent of all water pumped by the end of 1908. By the following year the figure had jumped to 87 percent. Problems developed in pumping water from Torresdale to high elevations in the Queen Lane district miles away in Northwest Philadelphia, and the city was forced to build another filtration plant on the Schuylkill. This meant more delay, but that facility was in operation on 1 November 1911. After a full year of city-wide filtration, the typhoid death rate was 13 per 100,000, the lowest since the city began to keep official typhoid records in 1861. By 1915 the death rate was down even further, to 7 per 100,000.

Despite all the progress, the city was not yet completely safe from typhoid because the disease was still a problem in rural areas and Philadelphians could contract it there and come home infected. In the summer of 1915 some Italian immigrants who were working on suburban farms as pickers drank contaminated water and became ill. When they returned home to Philadelphia, they infected their families, who unknowingly spread infection to the community when they went food shopping at the local greengrocer carts. Not all the produce they touched necessarily became contaminated, but apparently enough of it did to help spread the disease through the neighborhood.

To support its view that food infection and not the city's water was the villain, the board of health noted that 90 percent of the cases in the wards worst hit were among Italians while the incidence of typhoid was low among Jews, who also lived in large numbers in the same wards and drank the same water. The difference, said the health department, was because Italians liked to eat fresh salads and raw vegetables while the Jews cooked nearly everything, their religious practices thus acting as an effective if unintended prophylactic. In any event, the health department felt it safe to say that the city's water supply was "free from suspicion," a statement that seems accurate in light of the evidence.[17] Even with some continued contamination from outside sources, the death rate from typhoid was down to 5 per 100,000 by 1919 and by the early 1920s it was less than 1 per 100,000. This meant for all practical purposes Philadelphia had conquered typhoid, a happy phenomenon which was true by then in nearly all American cities.

The addition of chlorine to the water supply also helped to cut the death rate from typhoid during these years. Philadelphia first used it in 1909 as a way of treating the raw water still being used in the Queen Lane district and the results were so successful that from 1912 on chlorine was used as an additive for water in the entire system. Philadelphia was not the only city to use chlorine, nor the first, Jersey City being the first municipality to add it to its water supply in 1907 and years of experimental testing in several cities dated back to the 1890s.[18] Chlorine in fact was found to be such a powerful bactericide that Chicago for years was able to rely exclusively on the chemical alone and did not build filtration plants until 1947.[19]

Given the magic of chlorine, it might appear that Philadelphia wasted money by building filtration plants, but this was not the case because the only cities that were able to use the chemical without filters were those which had clear water—or made their water clearer, as Chicago had done in the early 1900s when it completed its sanitary canal that helped to keep sewerage away from Lake Michigan. On the other hand, chlorine did not work well in waters that were

---

[17]Board of Health, *Annual Report* (1915), 156-157. Shell fish taken from polluted waters are also a threat.
[18]Ravenel, ed., *A Half Century of Public Health*, 172-173.
[19]Louis P. Cain, *Sanitary Strategy for a Lakefront Metropolis* (DeKalb, Ill., 1978), 127.

frequently filled with sediment because dirt particles ab-
sorbed the chemical and limited its effectiveness. The
Schuylkill and Delaware fell into this category particularly in
rainy weather or when snow melted.

Dirt in the Schuylkill in fact was such a problem that the
water bureau was forced to build preliminary filters at
Lower Roxborough, Queen Lane, Belmont and Torresdale
in order to keep their main filters from clogging up too
quickly and lowering pumping efficiency. (The reservoir at
Upper Roxborough did not need one because water sat
there long enough for sedimentation to do a good enough
job.) The first "scrubber" as the pre-filters were called was
added to the Lower Roxborough filter a few years after it
began operation. It was so successful that more were built.

The scrubbers added $2.2 million to the costs of the filtra-
tion program, according to Ashbridge, who estimated in
1903 that the total costs of the improvements would be some
$26 million, a sum nearly double the $14.6 million estimate
of the experts in 1899. This seems like an extravagant increase, but the figure the experts provided is not a particularly accurate one because they were planning a system
that would be filtering only 200 million gallons a day, which
required a good deal less in the way of filters, pumps, and
pipes than a system that was filtering 300 million gallons
daily.

According to Ashbridge, the experts also made some er-
rors in their estimate by omitting the cost of an improvement
they recommended ($1 million for a distributing reservoir
near Olneyville), and by not including $500,000 for an addi-
tion to the reservoir at George's Hill in West Philadelphia.
The latter improvement was not on the experts' list, but
Ashbridge said it was necessary in order to implement their
filtration plans for that section of the city, so "in fairness," he
said, the sum "should be added to the experts' summary."[20]
In other words, according to Ashbridge, the estimate should
have been $17.2 million, and given the rising costs of mate-
rials and labor, he said a really accurate estimate for a system
filtering 200 million gallons daily would be a $21.6 million.

---

[20]Fourth Annual Message of Samuel Ashbridge in Bureau of Water *Annual Report*
(1902), xxvi.

This made the $26 million price tag for a 300 million gallon system look even better because, as Ashbridge pointed out, the city would be getting a 50 percent increase in filtered water with only a 30 percent increase in cost. Ashbridge compared the cost of Philadelphia's improvements with those in Boston, Cincinnati, St. Louis, New York, and San Francisco. He showed that Philadelphia was getting good value for its dollar, Boston, for example, then spending $19 million for work that would add only an extra 110 million gallons daily.[21]

By January of 1912 when the entire city of Philadelphia was receiving filtered water, the water bureau said the total costs of the improvements were $28 million, a figure higher than the estimate of Hill and Ashbridge, to be sure, but remarkably close considering how final costs have a tendency to balloon in construction projects. Indeed the final figures actually might be closer to $26 million than $28 million because the figures seem to include annual bureau salaries and wages for the period, and some of those costs would have been incurred even if the improvements had not taken place.[22]

What about graft? Undoubtedly there was some, but it is hard to say how much. When the McNichol brothers were challenged in 1905, they had an auditing firm inspect their contract books and corroborate their claim that they had not made excessive profits—and then give the audit report to the press.[23] To be sure, accountants could juggle the books a variety of ways to hide profits, as critics were quick to point out. But Gillette and Maclennan had not produced any evidence of wrong-doing and no follow-up reports were forthcoming, despite the first report having been called "preliminary."

According to an article in *World's Work*, the McNichols made $75,000 profit on a $290,000 contract for sand for the Torresdale filters when they sublet the contract to another firm for $215,000.[24] No doubt there was something in the

[21]Ibid., xxxiii-iv.
[22]Bureau of Water, *Annual Report* (1911), 30-31.
[23]*Inquirer*, 31 October 1905.
[24]Isaac F. Marcasson, "The Awakening of Philadelphia," *World's Work* 10 (Sept. 1905): 6647.

charge, but crooked contractors do not necessarily mean that city officials who awarded the contracts were crooks too. In any case, it is worth keeping the $28 million spent in Philadelphia in perspective, considering that the total costs of Chicago's sanitary canal ran to over $100 million, and New York spent some $188 million between 1905 and the late 1920s when it extended its watershed system into the Catskill Mountains.[25]

In an article in *McClure's* magazine in 1905 on "Typhoid: An Unnecessary Evil," Pittsburgh was called the "Home of Typhoid" for heading the list of American cities with the highest rate of cases per capita. It was building its own filtration plant, but taxpayers were not convinced it would work, the article said. "What guarantee is there that filtration of Pittsburgh water will save lives and suffering? One need look no further than Philadelphia for the answer."[26]

The previous year Philadelphia had been treated with a good deal less respect in another article that appeared in *McClure's*. This was the "corrupt and contented" article by Lincoln Steffens, which was reprinted in *The Shame of the Cities*. Philadelphia was run by a Republican machine, he said, that like a banyan tree "sends its roots from the center out both up and down and all around." Philadelphians were "supine," "asleep" and "hopelessly boss ruled."[27]

Steffens believed that corrupt businessmen were responsible for Philadelphia's problems, a view Steffens shared with Clinton Woodruff who was his local contact when Steffens visited the city to do his research. The businessmen bribed

[25]Cain, *Sanitation Strategy*, 80; Charles H. Weidner, *Water for a City; The History of New York City's Problem from the Beginning to the Delaware River System* (New Brunswick, N.J., 1974), 283.

[26]Samuel Hopkins Adams, "Typhoid," *McClure's* 25 (June 1905), 147. By the early 1900s the suburbs also enjoyed safe water supplied in large part by the Philadelphia Suburban Water Company, which bought many smaller companies and consolidated their operations. The company drew its water from clean upcountry streams and artesian wells. By the 1920s (and perhaps earlier) chlorine was added. For a brief history of the company, see Jerry A. Sacchetti ed., *Reflections on Water: A Centennial History of the Philadelphia Suburban Water Company* (Bryn Mawr, 1986).

[27]Steffens, *The Shame of the Cities*, 134, 143. On boss rule, Steffens says Ashbridge retired from office rich as a result of graft, but he supplies no evidence besides allegations of shakedowns. In any event, Ashbridge the Crook continues to be the standard view. See, for example, the entry in Melvin Holli and Peter d'A. Jones, eds., *Biographical Dictionary of American Mayors, 1820-1980* (Westport, Conn., 1981), 10. Steffen's article is cited as a source.

the politicians who in turn duped the voters—Steffens had first used this explanation of municipal corruption in an article in *Ainslee's* in 1901. The following year he joined *McClure's* and began writing the series that became *The Shame of the Cities*. In every city he visited Steffens found the same sordid relationship between politicians and businessmen. This strengthened his thesis, but it weakened the distinctiveness of Philadelphia's "corrupt and contented" image since the city seemed the same as others so far as its politics were concerned. In any event, Steffens was right that the Republicans ran Philadelphia, but he exaggerated a bit about civic apathy.

Note on Sources

This study relied heavily on the city's published records and contemporary newspapers in large part because the other sources are scarce. There are only a few scattered files of the relevant agencies for the period in the City Archives. The John Welsh collection in the Historical Society of Pennsylvania has some material on the cholera scare of 1892 but nothing on typhoid; the papers of William Pepper in the University of Pennsylvania library have some of his correspondence in the 1890s, but they do not include letters related to water reform that are cited in a biography of Pepper written by Francis Newton Thorpe in 1904. At the time Thorpe wrote his biography, the papers were in the possession of the Pepper family (Pepper died in 1898). Unfortunately sometime before the university received the papers, the letters were lost. The papers of Frank J. Firth in the Germantown Historical Society library are a valuable collection that fortunately has survived. Firth was a leader in the filtration movement, and the collection includes minutes of the City Organization's Filtration Committee (in existence from 1896 to 1902), copies of his correspondence as president, a scrapbook of newspaper clippings, and many pamphlets on filtration.

Some useful references on the politics of public health in other cities are Barbara Gutmann Rosenkrantz, *Public Health and the State: Changing Views in Massachusetts, 1842-1936* (Cambridge, Mass., 1972); Stuart Galishoff, *Safeguarding the Public Health, Newark, 1895-1918* (Westport, Conn., 1975); Martin V. Melosi, ed., *Pollution and Reform in American Cities, 1870-1930* (Austin, Texas, 1980); and Judith Walzer Leavitt,

The Healthiest City: Milwaukee and the Politics of Health Reform (Princeton, 1982). The best introduction to the field of public health, broadly viewed, is William H. McNeill, *Plagues and People* (Garden City, N.Y., 1976), an imaginative study that explores the impact of disease on world history from ancient times to the present.

Index

Aqueduct: proposed for Philadelphia, 9; in other cities, 7-9

Ashbridge, Samuel H.: biographical sketch, 62; role in 1899 mayoral election, 64-66; leadership assessed, 82-83

Bringhurst, Robert R.: biographical sketch, 70; role in Schuylkill Valley Water Company episode, 51; opposes Quaker Ciy Water Company bill, 67-68; view on filtration, 70-71

Cholera: described, 24; preventive measures in 1892, 25-27

Chlorine: as additive to water in Philadelphia and other cities, 93

City Organizations' Filtration Committee: and reform efforts, 37, 41, 47, 52, 73

Delaware River: pollution in, 7, 13-14

Filters: types, 32-33; in Lawrence, Mass., 23, 32; in London, 17; in Albany, N.Y., 43

Firth, Frank J. See City Organizations' Filtration Committee and Note on Sources

Graham, George S.: as prosecutor, 49-51; defends John Hill, 87

Green, Nelson: as lobbyist, 51-52, 66

Hazen, Allen: on water waste, 66

Hering, Rudolph: as consultant, 9, 79

Hill, John: as head of bureau of filtration, 86-87. See also Torresdale conduit

Lower Merion Township, Pa.: contributes to pollution problem in Schuylkill river, 51-52

Ludlow, William: comments on river pollution in 1883, 6-7; doubts about aqueduct water, 13

McNeil, William H.: quoted, 24

McNichol, Daniel and James: and construction controversies, 87-89, 95

Martin, David. See Philadelphia: mayoral elections and issues

Meehan, Thomas: biographical sketch, 33-34; opposes filtration, 34-39

Penrose, Boies. See Philadelphia: mayoral elections and issues, 1895

Pepper, William: as civic leader, 28, 42, 52

Philadelphia: mayoral elections and issues: in 1895, 18-22; in 1899, 62-66; in 1903, 86

Pine Barrens, N.J.: as possible water source, 44-46

Quaker City Water Company: bill for, 66-68

Schuylkill River: and pollution, 6-7, 54-55; and sewers, 14; water tests for, 10-12

Schuylkill Valley Water Company: bill for, 46-47; and bribery charges, 51-52

Sedimentation: as planning strategy, 14-15; Trautwine's views on, 30, 35

Steffens, Lincoln: views on Philadelphia, 3, 96-97

Torresdale conduit: described, 88-89; controversy over, 90-92

Trautwine, John C., Jr.: biographical sketch, 29-30; and meters, 31-32, 58-61, 77, 82-83, 91-92; requests for filters, 32, 58-59; dispute with councilmen in 1896, 33-39; and Torresdale conduit, 91-92

Typhoid: causes, 1; epidemics in Philadelphia: in 1897-98, 53-54; in 1899, 1-3, 69-70; in 1906, 85; in 1915, 92-93

Warner, Sam B., Jr.: quoted, 3; on 1906 epidemic, 85 fn

Warwick, Charles F.: biographical sketch, 21-22; role as mayor assessed, 76-77. See also Philadelphia: mayoral elections and issues, 1895

Well water: in Philadelphia, 56-57

Wharton, Joseph. See Pine Barrens, N.J.

Woman's Health Protective Association: and reform, 22, 36, 41, 43, 52

Woodruff, Clinton Rogers: and views, 84, 96

www.ingramcontent.com/pod-product-compliance
Lightning Source LLC
Chambersburg PA
CBHW021109290326
41932CB00040BA/1